COPING WITH
Osteoarthritis

COPING WITH
Osteoarthritis

Sound, Compassionate Advice
for People Dealing with the Challenge
of Osteoarthritis

ROBERT H. PHILLIPS, PH.D.

Avery
A MEMBER OF
PENGUIN PUTNAM INC.
NEW YORK

Most Avery books are available at special quantity discounts for bulk purchase for sales promotions, premiums, fund-raising, and educational needs. Special books or book excerpts also can be created to fit specific needs. For details, write Putnam Special Markets, 375 Hudson Street, New York, NY 10014.

a member of
Penguin Putnam Inc.
375 Hudson Street
New York, NY 10014
www.penguinputnam.com

Library of Congress Cataloging-in-Publication Data
Phillips, Robert H., date.
Coping with osteoarthritis : sound, compassionate advice for
people dealing with the challenges of osteoarthritis / Robert H. Phillips.
p.   cm.
Includes bibliographical references and index.
ISBN 1-58333-090-9
1. Osteoarthritis—Popular Works.   2. Osteoarthritis—Psychological aspects.   3. Adjustment (Psychology).   I. Title.

RC931.O67P45   2001   00-048540
616.7'223—dc21

Printed in the United States of America
1   3   5   7   9   8   6   4   2

Book design by Jennifer Ann Daddio

Contents

PART THREE
Your Emotions

PART FOUR
Interacting with Other People

This book is lovingly dedicated to my family—
my wife, Sharon, and my three sons,
Michael, Larry, and Steven;
my daughter-in-law Donna and her family;
my parents, sister, mother-in-law, nephews, niece, and favorite aunt;
and all my other relatives and in-laws—and to my friends.

Acknowledgments

I'd like to express appreciative words of thanks to some wonderful people who provided valuable assistance in the preparation of the original edition of this book, as well as this new one. Thanks to Robert Marcus, M.D., and Richard Furie, M.D., for their critical reviews, helpful suggestions and information, and support for this project. Thanks to William Given, M.D., for his insightful review of the manuscript. Thanks to Sharon Balaban (first edition) and Kathy Green (second edition) for the hours spent painstakingly transcribing, revising, and typing the final manuscript. Finally, grateful thanks to Roland Moskowitz, M.D., for a professional evaluation of the highest caliber.

Foreword

Osteoarthritis (OA), also known as degenerative joint disease, is the most common form of arthritis, affecting 20 million or more Americans. Many people (including, at times, physicians!) look at osteoarthritis as a "nuisance" that causes some mild aches and pains but never really incapacitates people. Unfortunately, in many individuals it is more than a minor problem and can lead to significant pain, limitation, and overall disability, particularly when it involves significant joints such as the hips, knees, or spine. The enormity of the problem posed by osteoarthritis is seen in the statistics, which show that after age 70, up to 85 percent of the general population has evidence of this disorder; in approximately 25 percent of these cases, the symptoms may be severe enough to require some form of treatment. Another common misconception is that little can be done to relieve osteoarthritis symptoms and that seeking help is without benefit. On the contrary, much can be done in the way of symptomatic relief; at times, joint protection may slow down the disease process.

Dr. Phillips has written an admirable book on how to cope with the disease. In order to cope successfully, you have to understand what the disorder is; this is outlined with clarity in sections describing what the disease is, how it is diagnosed, and how it is treated. Important questions, such as how pain can be handled, what effects special diets do (or do not) have, and when exercise or rest is appropriate, are all considered in a balanced fashion. Other sections deal with how patients and families handle the disease and how someone with OA can lead a healthy, wholesome existence while still not ignoring the important do's of management.

Chronic diseases are tough to handle—nobody teaches us how to do this while we're growing up. Dr. Phillips has put together a volume replete with understanding, sensitivity, and humor. He provides a commonsense approach to managing and coping with this disorder that, if followed, will reduce its impact on everyday life. What you can do, not what you can't do, is stressed. (Life has enough don'ts without adding to them unnecessarily.) The concepts can be carried over to other stresses in everyday life. I look forward to recommending this volume to my many patients with this disorder.

—Roland W. Moskowitz, M.D.
Professor of Medicine,
Case Western Reserve University
Director, Division of Rheumatic Diseases,
University Hospitals of Cleveland

Preface

Osteoarthritis can certainly have an impact on you and your family—make no bones about it! When you are diagnosed, many questions may come to mind. Physicians or other professionals can answer some of them. You may find answers in other books or articles on the subject. There is also a wealth of information on the Internet. However, many questions still remain, because experts just don't have all the answers. And this can be frustrating and upsetting. It can also be upsetting to realize that this is happening to *you*. Living with osteoarthritis can be depressing unless you learn how to think positively and make necessary changes.

Fortunately, medical science has made a great deal of progress in treating and controlling osteoarthritis, and continues to make progress. So there is every chance that you will be able to lead a normal and productive life. But what about the psychological effects of osteoarthritis? Will it interfere with your lifestyle? Will you be able to handle the pain? A major factor in determining your potential to lead a normal, emotionally stable life is how well you cope with osteoarthritis.

Powerful stuff? It certainly is, but that's why this book was written! It's filled with information, suggestions, and strategies to help you, your family, and your friends learn how to cope successfully with osteoarthritis.

This is the second edition of *Coping with Osteoarthritis*. The first edition was published in 1989, and the response to it was extremely gratifying. Since that time, there have been some important new developments in our understanding of and ability to manage osteoarthritis that have made an update necessary—hence this second edition. The first part of this book presents basic information about the disease: what it is, what the symptoms are, and what treatments are available. The remainder of the book deals with everyday challenges, including coping with emotions, making lifestyle changes, and dealing with other people. We will explore each aspect in detail, examine many suggestions and strategies, and look at real-life examples. In fact, a lot of the information you will read can—and does—apply to any chronic medical condition. This book, however, focuses specifically on your life with osteoarthritis.

As you learn to cope with this disease, it is important to realize that you are not alone; millions of others and their families and friends are experiencing many of the same struggles and emotions as you. This can be very reassuring. Remember, though, that each person is unique, so symptoms will vary and response to treatment can be different. What works well for one may not work at all for another. Similarly, the psychological consequences of having osteoarthritis can be difficult. Your life with this disease—the way it affects you and the way you react to it—will not be the same as anyone else's. Therefore, it will be up to *you* to use the suggestions and strategies presented in this book to help yourself cope as well as you possibly can. This book was written to help you take charge of your body and become an active, rather than a passive, participant in your treatment plan.

Researchers are working hard trying to find a cure for osteoarthritis. But until they do, you will have to learn to live with it. I hope this book will help both you and your family to do just that, and to do it comfortably and while feeling in control.

—Robert H. Phillips, Ph.D.
Center for Coping
Long Island, N.Y.

PART ONE

Osteoarthritis:
An Overview

CHAPTER ONE

What Is Osteoarthritis?

Eleanor, a 59-year-old account executive, had been feeling achy and uncomfortable for quite a while. Recently, however, she had begun to notice that her pain seemed to linger longer than before. In the past, she had chosen to just live with it. But now, with pain affecting her knees, hips, and finger joints, it hurt to even move. Finally, she took time off from work and dragged herself (painfully!) to the doctor. She told him that she had to know what was going on, because the pain just wasn't getting any better. The doctor performed a complete physical examination, a number of blood tests, and a series of x-rays. After analyzing all the results, he sat Eleanor down and said, "Well, it's osteoarthritis, but at least now your pain has a name." Eleanor's resigned reaction was "So what do I do now?"

Yes, Eleanor had osteoarthritis (OA), one of more than a hundred different types of arthritis, all of which affect the joints of the body. The major forms of arthritis can be divided into two main categories—inflammatory or degenerative—depending on how the joints are damaged. OA is in the degenerative category—it is a chronic degenerative disease. Why is it called *degenerative*? Because it occurs when, for some reason, the cartilage (the smooth cushion that lines the ends of the bones) degenerates, or wears down. This allows the bones to come closer together, which causes a narrowing of the joint space that can be seen in x-rays. As a result, the bones in the joint rub together when you move. This can be painful. In addition, when cartilage covering bone breaks down and the bones grind together, the body may respond by thickening the end of the bone. Additional bone formations, also called osteophytes or bone spurs, may compound the problem and add to the pain.

The prefix *osteo* means "bone," *arthr(o)* means "joints," and *itis* means inflammation. Thus, *osteoarthritis* literally means "inflammation of the bones in a joint." But this is not a totally accurate description of the condition, so osteoarthritis is also called *osteoarthrosis* (a disease or condition affecting bones in a joint) or *degenerative joint disease* (DJD).

In order to better understand OA, let's talk a little bit about the body parts most affected by this disease.

Welcome to the Joint!

"The anklebone's connected to the shinbone; the shinbone's connected to the kneebone; the kneebone's connected to the thighbone . . ." and so on. You may recognize these lines as the lyrics to an old spiritual. But they're not anatomically correct! The bones are *not* directly connected to each other. Rather, tendons, ligaments, and muscles connect them. An area where two or more bones come together forms what we know as a joint (also called an *articulation*), and is enclosed in a covering called the joint capsule.

What is the joint for? It permits motion. So it is a very important structure. Why? It does a lot of hard work. Stop and think for a moment about the millions of times you move different joints in your body each day. Just today you've probably already yawned, stretched, stood up, or sat down. In addition, every time you move, it's rarely one simple joint that's moving. Usually, a number of joints are involved in any one movement. Think about how much wear and tear each of your joints will experience in your lifetime. It is remarkable to think that, for the most part, joint movement is smooth, frictionless, and painless.

Let us now look at the anatomy of the joint as it relates to osteoarthritis. Not all joints are structured in exactly the same way, nor is it necessary to go into detail concerning every single structure of the joint. This discussion will focus on and emphasize the structures that are important in osteoarthritis.

CARTILAGE

Picture the ends of two bones that meet at a joint. They need protection so that they won't keep banging against each other, wearing each other out. So the end of each bone is covered by a smooth, white, firm, rubbery, connective tissue, up to one-eighth inch thick, called cartilage. The cartilage creates smooth, elastic, resilient surfaces that can rub against each other with very little friction, especially when properly lubricated. What does the lubricating? No, not your local gas-station mechanic. The cartilage is kept wet and moving smoothly by a substance called *synovial fluid*. The synovial membrane, which lines the tough, fibrous joint capsule surrounding each joint, produces this fluid.

Cartilage acts as a shock absorber within the joint. One of the four layers in joint cartilage is composed primarily of complex molecules called *proteoglycans*. Proteoglycans in cartilage are arranged in a structure that holds fluid when the joint is at rest, much as a sponge can hold water. When the joint is used, and the bones press together, the fluid is pressed out into the joint space. Then, when the joint relaxes again, the proteoglycans reabsorb the fluid, restoring the normal shape of the cartilage and preparing the joint for its next use.

Cartilage and bone tissue are both constantly in the process of being regenerated—old cartilage and bone are broken down and replaced with newly manufactured tissue. Normally, all parts of the joint (such as the bone, cartilage, and synovial fluid) are present in the right quantities and work smoothly together. But if they don't . . . ouch!

TYPES OF JOINTS

The joints in the human body can be grouped into three categories, depending on the kind and degree of movement they allow. The first category is the *immovable joint*. The joints of the skull are one example. The bones of the skull fit together in an interlocking pattern to protect the brain. It is not necessary to consider the immovable joints as part of our discussion of osteoarthritis.

The second type of joint is the *slightly movable joint*. The joints in this category do not move very much, but there is a little bit of flexibility built into the joint structure. Examples of slightly movable joints are the vertebrae—the bones of the spinal column. The cartilage protecting them forms cushiony pads called *intervetebral discs*. Osteoarthritis can affect these joints.

The third type of joint is the *movable joint*. Examples include the joints of the fingers, toes, hips, ankles, and knees. These are the joints people usually refer to when they casually talk about their joints. They are also the ones that may be primarily involved in osteoarthritis.

What Causes OA?

In discussing the causes of OA, it is important to begin with the two main classifications of the disease: primary and secondary.

Primary osteoarthritis (also called *idiopathic osteoarthritis*) refers to the condition that develops for no apparent reason, other than possibly age or "wear and tear" (a description that is not totally accurate, by the way).

Secondary osteoarthritis, on the other hand, usually has more specific underlying influences. You've read, for example, about athletes who have had to retire because of the joint damage that was suffered from years of sports activities. In extreme cases, people whose work (or play) puts prolonged, intense, excessive pressure on the joints may develop secondary osteoarthritis. Secondary osteoarthritis can occur some time after the occurrence of any number of precipitating factors, including traumatic injury (such as a fracture); problems with a joint (such as infection or congenital deformities); or repeated stress to a joint (such as that experienced by athletes, ballet dancers, and even typists, among others). Another disease, such as rheumatoid arthritis, can damage a joint and lead to osteoarthritis as well as rheumatoid arthritis in the same joint (double ouch!). Being overweight can contribute to the development of secondary osteoarthritis. If you are overweight, you are placing added pounds of pressure on your weight-bearing joints!

Although the exact underlying cause of OA is still unknown, much knowledge about OA has been gained through research. There are a number of factors that may play a role in the development of the disease, although that doesn't mean that any of these factors actually *cause* osteoarthritis. Examples include:

- Age (the incidence of osteoarthritis increases dramatically after age forty-five to fifty).
- Gender (for example, women are more likely to develop OA of the hands).
- Lack of exercise (exercise is necessary for joint flexibility and maintained muscle strength).
- Overweight (extra pounds mean added stress on weight-bearing joints).
- Occupational or recreational strain (more intense, physical activities can increase risk).
- Overuse or injuries to joints (trauma to a joint increases the likelihood of developing OA in that joint, especially if proper healing did not occur).
- Hereditary conditions (for example, defective cartilage or malformation of a joint increases the likelihood of developing OA).

One perplexing question continues to be why some people seem to be more vulnerable to the onset and progression of OA than others. In some cases, there may be a genetic component—a faulty gene responsible for the production of certain components of cartilage. Metabolic and hormonal factors may be involved as well. Recent research suggests that in some people, problems within the structure of the cartilage may be at the root of osteoarthritis. Specifically, the cartilage in the joints may become supersaturated, which eventually weakens it and leads to erosion of the cartilage. Why this happens is not clear, however.

How Does OA Occur?

Unlike other chronic diseases, OA has a fairly typical pattern of symptoms. Regardless of whether you have primary or secondary osteoarthritis, or which specific joints are affected, the destruction of cartilage and resulting overgrowth of bone spurs usually occur in a similar manner. The one varying factor is how far these cartilage and bone changes will go.

In most cases, the onset of osteoarthritis is fairly slow. Often, OA may be noticed on an x-ray—without the person ever having had pain or injury. It may take many months, but usually takes years, for cartilage to wear down to the point that pain occurs. But even then, there is a lot of variability in the way people experience OA pain. It can range from mild to seemingly constant pain, or there may be times when you don't hurt at all. Fortunately, in the majority of cases, pain rarely exceeds a moderate level. When it does, it is usually only after you have strenuously exerted yourself. In a smaller percentage of cases, OA can progress to the point of more intense, constant pain. Joints can sometimes be seriously affected, leading to deformity and significantly reduced mobility. It is virtually impossible to predict to what degree osteoarthritis will develop in different people.

Who Gets OA?

If you have osteoarthritis, you are certainly not alone. OA is a very common disease. It is estimated that in the United States alone, tens of millions of people have osteoarthritis. And although most people have some form of OA by the time they are in their sixties or seventies, in many cases their OA is detected only by x-ray. And x-ray abnormalities may not correlate with symptoms. A person whose x-rays show the presence of OA may not experience any symptoms, or any symptoms they do experience may be mild enough to be "handle-able." But osteoarthritis is not just a "senior's" disease. Some people develop OA in their forties and fifties, some at even younger ages, especially if there are specific secondary causes for the onset of the disease.

Considering all age groups, there seems to be a fairly equal number of men and women with OA. However, among people under age forty-five, OA is more common in men, while in people over fifty-five, the incidence is higher in women. This may be because secondary OA, which often begins earlier in life than primary OA, is more prevalent in men. Primary OA is much more common in women, and its incidence increases with age.

Some people believe that where you live may affect your likelihood of developing OA. And some studies have suggested that osteoarthritis is less prevalent in more northerly regions. But, in fact, there is no specific geographic location whose inhabitants are more or less prone to osteoarthritis. Individuals in all parts of the world can and do develop OA.

Climate also seems to be of little importance. You might prefer living in a certain type of climate, and you may notice that you may feel more or less comfortable in different climates, but research has not shown that any type of climate plays a significant role in the development or progression of osteoarthritis.

What Joints Are Affected?

Osteoarthritis seems to affect certain joints more than others. The hands and knees seem to be affected the most. The hips, feet, and spine also are often affected.

Let's talk about your hands for a moment. Each of your fingers has three joints: the base, the middle knuckle, and the distal joint (the small joint near the end or tip of the finger). Osteoarthritis is far more likely to affect the distal and middle joints than the base joint, although base joints can occasionally be affected also, especially in the thumbs. If OA spurs develop on the distal joints of your fingers, the bumps that result are called *Heberden's nodes.* If they develop on or affect the knuckles, the bumps are called *Bouchard's nodes.*

In addition to affecting the hands, osteoarthritis usually affects weight-bearing joints. This is one reason the knees and the hips are frequently involved. The feet and toes frequently develop OA—especially the big toe. The spine is affected as well, both the cervical spine (the neck region) and the lumbar spine (the lower back region). Damage can affect the intervertebral discs, which serve as the shock absorbers, keeping the bones separated and comfortably cushioned, or bone spurs can grow on the vertebrae themselves. Spurs can pinch nerves or can narrow the spinal canal, a condition known as *spinal stenosis,* and can even pinch the spinal cord itself.

Often, joints of the body become affected symmetrically, such as both hips or both knees being involved. But in some cases, only a few joints may be affected, and asymmetrically.

Although other joints, including shoulders and ankles, may be affected by osteoarthritis, this occurs only rarely. Shoulder pain is very common, but the pain usually arises from problems with the rotator cuff tendons as opposed to disorders of the joint. Primary OA usually affects finger joints first, then the big toes, and then one or more of the weight-bearing joints, such as the hips and knees. Part of the spine may also be affected by primary OA. Secondary OA rarely affects more than a few joints, and often affects only one or two joints. Most often, secondary OA affects the hips, knees, ankles, or big toes. Why? Because these are the primary weight-bearing joints of the body—the ones that are most apt to be injured.

Muscles also can be affected in OA. They seem to get tired and are unable to work as hard as they used to. This can be a problem, since strong muscles support joints and help them move. If joints are painful because of cartilage degeneration, muscles have to work harder to support joint movement. Weakened muscles cannot help the joints as much. Also, weak muscles can lead to an unstable joint, one that wobbles. This can cause even more wear and tear, leading to more degeneration. The joint and muscle problems of OA can cause a vicious cycle of discomfort and reduced mobility.

What Are the Symptoms and Signs?

OA causes both symptoms and signs. What's the difference? Simply put, symptoms are what you feel and signs are things your doctor can observe. Now that we've gotten that out of the way, let's talk about what what happens with OA.

Symptoms and manifestations of osteoarthritis vary from person to person. What is the primary symptom of OA? Pain! It may begin as stiffness, soreness, or an aching sensation. In early stages, pain is felt when moving or shortly afterward. Activity tends to increase the amount of pain you feel. Fortunately, rest can relieve this pain, although stiffness can result from resting. (Sometimes it may seem like you just can't win!) In more advanced OA, you may experience pain even if you're resting. It may become so intense that it hurts to even exercise the affected joints. Pain is an essential barometer in determining how OA is affecting you.

In addition to pain, other problems do occasionally occur. A noticeable sign of progressing OA is reduced mobility. You may find you just can't move the way you used to. Why? As cartilage in certain joints breaks down, you'll experience more pain from joint movement. Reduced joint mobility occurs as you instinctively limit your movements to avoid pain, combined with a narrowing of the joint spaces, weaker muscles, bone spurs, or fragments of bone and cartilage in your joints. In arthritis that affects the spine, if bone spurs from one vertebra grow to become fused with the next higher or lower vertebra, a significant loss of flexibility will occur.

Other signs of OA include crepitus (a crackling or grating noise heard or felt in moving joints) and joint enlargement (due to bone changes). Heberden's nodes and Bouchard's nodes (see page 9) are other trademarks of OA.

In some cases, inflammation can occur in osteoarthritis, but it is usually mild. This may contribute to the pain or tenderness you notice when the joint is touched. Significant inflammation is generally detected only in a relatively uncommon form of OA called *inflammatory* or *erosive OA*. This condition has certain similarities to rheumatoid arthritis (RA), and it is best to see a rheumatologist for the diagnosis and treatment of it.

Unlike some other forms of arthritis, OA doesn't affect organs of the body, such as the heart, kidneys, or lungs. And other common signs of illness, such as fever, changes in appetite, or feelings of malaise, are not as much a factor as they might be in inflammatory types of arthritis such as rheumatoid arthritis.

How Is OA Diagnosed?

To accurately diagnose OA, your doctor may use any of a number of methods, including a complete medical history, a physical examination, and x-rays. Blood and laboratory tests also may be employed. The latter are usually done not to diagnose OA directly, but to rule out other forms of arthritis or other diseases as the cause of symptoms.

Listening to the individual's description of his or her current symptoms and examining the joints are the most important parts of the evaluation. X-rays are usually required to confirm the physician's diagnosis and to determine how severe the OA is.

MEDICAL HISTORY

The first step in diagnosing osteoarthritis is for your doctor to get a detailed medical history from you. To get a clear picture of just what you have been experiencing, and why, your doctor will likely ask a series of questions, such as:

- Where are the aches and pains?
- Which joints hurt?
- How long have they hurt?
- What time of day do they bother you the most?
- What seems to help?
- Do you experience any stiffness? If so, under what circumstances, and how long does it last?
- What injuries have you experienced to your joints?

These are just some of the many questions that may be asked. You may also be asked for information about the types of work you have done and what it involved; hobbies or other leisure activities you have engaged in; and whether other family members have a history of OA. These are all important factors in arriving at a diagnosis.

PHYSICAL EXAMINATION

During your physical exam, the physician will try to determine your general state of health, as well as the health of your joints. Your physician will check your joints carefully, and will look for joints that show signs of tenderness, redness, warmth, swelling, or inflammation. Your doctor will look, touch, and listen for any kind of abnormality, and will carefully observe movement of your joints, focusing on any signs of crepitus (bones rubbing together within a joint). There may be a difference between the *active range of motion* of a joint (how far you can move a joint on your own) and the *passive range of motion* of the same joint (how far the doctor is able to move the joint). The doctor should also check your muscles for any signs of weakness or spasm. Finally, you will be examined for other specific signs of osteoarthritis, such as Heberden's nodes or Bouchard's nodes. If you have OA, your doctor should be able to diagnose it based on your history and the findings of your physical examination.

X-RAYS

X-rays can be an important assessment tool for OA. A number of bone changes that are characteristic of the disease can be visualized on x-rays, including bone spurs and narrowing of joint spaces. Early in the development of OA, x-rays may not clearly show any changes. So why bother? Well, there's still an advantage to taking early x-rays. They provide a baseline against which later x-rays can be compared to see whether the disease is advancing. They can also show doctors how well treatment programs are controlling the progression of the disease. They may alert the doctor to other problems that may be causing or contributing to your of pain, such as gout, osteonecrosis (death of bone cells due to an inadequate blood supply), Paget's disease (a bone disease that results in abnormally large but also abnormally fragile bones), or tumors. Normal x-rays in the presence of pain may signal a need for further evaluation with other imaging techniques, such as magnetic resonance imaging (MRI) or bone scans. X-rays can also determine if joint damage is severe enough that you might consider joint replacement surgery.

What exactly do doctors look for in x-rays? If cartilage is breaking down or has worn away in a joint, an x-ray can show a narrowing within the joint space. X-rays can show the formation of spurs or osteophytes (new bone growths that can contribute to the pain and restricted mobility of OA) and cysts. X-rays can even show bone fragments floating within the joint capsule, indicating degeneration. All of these findings, and others, can contribute to a diagnosis of OA, and can help to determine the severity of the problem.

What Is the Prognosis?

What is the prognosis for osteoarthritis? Unfortunately, it's hard to say. Doctors have a difficult time predicting how OA will affect any particular individual. Fortunately, most people with osteoarthritis can be prevented from experiencing serious pain and immobility, and can continue to live satisfying, productive lives.

Is there any way of predicting whether your OA will stay the same, get better, or even get worse? Unfortunately, no. But treatment does help. And the earlier you begin treatment for OA, and the more you comply with your prescribed treatment, the better the chances of helping yourself feel better.

Learn about your illness. If you learn about OA, you can deal with it better. Reading books and attending courses and seminars, among other activities, will help you to gain knowledge of OA. All these activities are offered by the Arthritis Foundation (see the Resources section of this book). Call your local chapter for information booklets or other Arthritis Foundation–related information. Don't be afraid to ask your doctor any questions that you have. If you are informed and educated, you'll even be able to assist your doctor in your care.

Other than your conscientious involvement, what is the most critical variable in how well you will fare with this condition? Proper treatment! Without it, osteoarthritis can get worse. But even if your OA doesn't get worse, not following proper treatment programs can lead to your condition becoming more painful that it needs to be. So the goal is to learn—and do—what you can! In the next chapter, we will look at the various ways in which OA is treated.

CHAPTER TWO

How Is Osteoarthritis Treated?

So far, we have discussed what OA is, who may get it, what the symptoms are, and how it is diagnosed, as well as other details about the disease. Terrific, but you're probably less concerned about what it is and where it came from than you are about how you can reduce your pain.

Some unhappy people fear that once they have OA, they can't do much to stop it from progressing into a severely crippling, deforming, and incapacitating illness. This couldn't be further from the truth. Sure, infrequently, OA can continue to progress despite all therapeutic efforts. However, in most cases, a good, comprehensive treatment program can help you to live a comfortable and satisfying (even if not totally pain-free) life.

So you probably have some important questions. What can your doctor do for you? What can you do for yourself? What are the different types of treatment for OA and how can they help you? How do you control your symptoms? How can you help yourself function better, with less pain? How do you determine the best treatment for *your* OA? Let's begin to answer some of your questions.

Each Person Is Unique

Before looking at any of the specifics of treatment, it is important to realize that your experience with OA is unique. No one else has exactly the same symptoms or reactions to the disease. So your treatment program will be unique as well, and specific to your own needs.

Each physician usually has his or her own ideas as to what approaches work best. A certain amount of trial and error may go into developing the best treatment plan for you, and you may even feel like a human guinea pig from time to time. But remember, this is only because the goal is to find the program that works best for *you*.

It is very important for you to feel at ease with your physician. You want to have confidence that the interventions prescribed for you will work. What if you heard that somebody else with OA was following a different program prescribed by another physician, and you started to believe that that treatment might be better? You might start losing confidence in your treatment plan, and then in your own physician. Not a great feeling, is it? Always remember, there is no one answer! What works for other people will not necessarily work for you.

The best treatment for OA can vary, depending on a number of factors, including your age, the severity of your OA, the extent of the pain, your lifestyle, and your personal preferences. A carefully structured, comprehensive treatment program can often be successful in controlling symptoms well enough that you can function quite well. However, there are times when some or all of the approaches may not be 100-percent successful or able to eliminate all of your pain. But you'll cross that bridge if and when you come to it.

So what should you do? Make sure you're seeing a doctor whom you can trust. (More about this in Chapter 23.) Then work closely with him or her, and with any other health-care professionals who are part of your treatment team. Because you might receive various forms of treatment at different times, it is important to be aware of all the options available for OA. Then make sure you fully understand your doctor's recommendations, and the rationale for them. Depending on your case, you may or may not be able to consider different options. If your situation *does* allow you to make choices, you will want to have the information you need to make the best possible decisions. If you don't understand or agree with your physician's treatment choices, consider getting another opinion. You want to make sure that you are getting the best, most appropriate, and potentially helpful treatment possible.

Treatment Goals

The ideal treatment outcome would be curing OA. But that's why treatment for OA can be so frustrating—there is no known cure for the disease. There is no pill that will stop the breakdown of cartilage. There is no surgical procedure that will eliminate the illness. There is no injection that will restore a joint to its original healthy condition—at least, not yet (although there is a lot of exciting research underway investigating how to restore cartilage or prevent its degeneration).

Since OA cannot be cured, it's better to consider your treatment program as more of a management program. As such, treatment ideally aims at a suppression of symptoms. You want to feel better, right? You want to live as normal a life as possible, don't you? So the main goal of treatment is to control your pain! Although no treatment is 100-percent effective in controlling *all* symptoms, hopefully treatment for OA will stabilize your condition. This is certainly a goal worth shooting for.

Keeping this in mind, what are the general goals of treatment? There are basically four:

1. To reduce or relieve pain.
2. To preserve function.
3. To maintain or increase strength and mobility, allowing you to keep your joints functioning as smoothly and as effectively as possible.
4. To prevent deformity, or prevent further damage if deformities have already occurred.

Planning Your Treatment

Treatment programs are usually developed by a team of health-care professionals, including physicians, mental-health professionals (psychiatrists, psychologists, and/or social workers, physical therapists (who treat disorders of the muscles, bones, or joints by using physical agents such as heat, cold, water, massage, and exercise), occupational therapists (who help people with physical problems through selected work and/or play activities to improve muscle strength, retrain them for employment, or help them relearn activities essential for daily living), and rehabilitation specialists (who treat individuals with disabilities by helping them to build on their strengths to improve their quality of life and ability to live independently). Initially, your primary-care physician may be the one most directly involved in planning your treatment program. Consultations with a rheumatologist (who may be your primary-care physician), orthopedic surgeon, or podiatrist may be advisable in some situations.

Components of Treatment Programs

Because OA can affect different people in different ways, each treatment program is individual and unique. Your own treatment program will depend on many factors. For example, how severe is your OA? How long have you had it? Which joints are affected? Other factors such as your age, overall general health, family situation, lifestyle, and occupation will also be taken into consideration.

Most treatment programs take a sensible, conservative approach, which is best for long-term results and your safety. Because there is no one particular treatment that is best for every person with OA, the program that you'll follow is a "package"—a combination of strategies. Your treatment program may include any or all of the following:

- Rest.
- Exercise.

- Medication (to control pain and reduce inflammation).
- Physical aids and other assistance devices.
- Physical therapy.
- Other methods to control pain and improve mobility.

Occasionally, surgery may be an adjunct to the treatment program. Any complete treatment program also attempts to help you deal with the emotional difficulties you may experience as a result of your OA, not just with the physical difficulties. In addition, many people find relief from complementary or alternative strategies. Finally, and very importantly, treatment programs may include modifications in your lifestyle. This chapter will provide an overview of these different components. More details on these subjects will be found later on in the book.

MEDICAL COMPONENTS

There are two main categories of conventional medical treatment for OA: medication and surgery. Each has its own particular role and uses.

Medication

Many different types of medication can be helpful for people with OA. Which medications are prescribed will vary, depending on the therapeutic goal. The most commonly used medications are painkillers, including acetaminophen (also sold under a variety of brand names, among them Tylenol, Datril, and others), aspirin, and nonsteroidal anti-inflammatory drugs (NSAIDs). Other types of medication also may be part of your treatment. (Specific medications will be covered in Chapter 6.)

Surgery

Most people with osteoarthritis never require surgery for it. If they do, they may benefit from relatively simple procedures such as arthroscopy (a procedure that may be used to "clean out" bone or cartilage fragments in a joint). However, in severe cases, surgical techniques such as replacement of the hip, knees, or shoulder joint have been successful in relieving pain and increasing mobility. As a result, many people have found surgery to be an important technique to improve quality of life. (More information on surgery can be found in Chapter 7.)

NONMEDICAL COMPONENTS

In addition to the medical components discussed above, there are a number of nonmedical measures you can use to help yourself as part of an overall treatment package. Stress management, exercise, proper nutrition, and various coping strategies can all be very helpful in improving both your physical and your emotional well-being.

Stress Management

Stress management is an important part of a comprehensive treatment program for dealing with OA. A number of different strategies can be employed to help you deal with both physiological and psychological stress. An important goal in stress management is to improve your feeling of being in control, in terms of both your emotions and your behavior, and to reduce pain-exacerbating tension. (Detailed information on stress and how to manage it can be found in Chapter 18.)

Exercise

Exercise is another important part of your treatment regimen. Exercise can help you feel better physically and can even reduce pain, as well as reducing stress and depression and enhancing self-esteem. It can also be very helpful in increasing general fitness, improving the way your body works, and enhancing the way you perceive your health. Different types of exercise may be used to help with various aspects of OA. Of course, all exercise should be performed only under medical supervision. (Exercise will be covered in detail in Chapter 9.)

Diet

Good nutrition is a powerful way to create health. Proper diet is an important part of comprehensive treatment for virtually any health problem. It is necessary to nourish your body and maintain as much strength and vitality as you can. The main dietary goals for OA is to maintain your body weight (or reduce it if you're overweight) and ensure a proper, balanced diet. (More information and specific recommendations regarding diet can be found in Chapter 8.)

Psychological Improvement

An important component of any treatment program for OA is successful coping. This means dealing effectively with the pain—as well as the ups and downs—of your condition, and maintaining a positive mental attitude. There are many techniques that can be used and practical things that can be done to achieve these goals. We will be looking at a number of them in more detail throughout the rest of the book.

COMPLEMENTARY/ALTERNATIVE STRATEGIES

A growing number of people are interested in learning more about alternative treatments, also sometimes called nontoxic therapies, complementary treatments, and nonconventional therapies—and, by critics, unorthodox approaches. Why this increasing interest? People with OA want to find the safest and most natural ways of treating this disease. They may want to use alternative therapies as a means of strengthening their bodies and controlling side effects while undergoing conventional treatment, or to complement conventional treatment. Some people simply prefer the gentler, noninvasive approach of alternative therapies that may have fewer side effects than conventional treatments.

Despite the fact that there are a number of different types of alternative treatments, they do have common themes. Many alternative therapies, for example, are based on the belief that a truly healthy body is much less vulnerable to conditions such as OA. All alternative methods are designed to create (or re-create) the healthiest body possible so as to reduce or eliminate the vulnerability that allowed the disease to develop in the first place. The hope is that a healthier body state will enhance the body's healing processes and reduce the progression and severity of OA and its symptoms.

Be aware that most alternative therapies have not been tested in rigid, scientific studies. In addition, little scientific research has been done to investigate how (or if) any of the substances used in alternative strategies are absorbed by the body, how they may affect body organs, or how they may interact with other medications.

So make sure that you use due diligence in learning about alternative therapies. You can learn about them from a number of sources. By visiting libraries and bookstores, contacting health organizations, and exploring web sites that focus on OA, you should be able to obtain up-to-date information both about your OA and about all available treatments.

Your Role in Treatment

Regardless of the components chosen for your treatment, you play the most important role of all. Remember that what may work for family members or friends may not work for you. There are always things that you can do to help yourself. It doesn't matter how much medical knowledge you have—and you can always learn more. There are also things you can do to make your condition worse that, obviously, are to be *avoided*. To start helping yourself, identify those things that improve your condition and those things that hurt it. Learning what treatment is best for you may take time. But it's time worth spending.

As you follow your treatment regimen, do your best to adhere to it completely and accurately and to be as active a participant as possible. Be alert to the progress you make, and keep an open mind. Feel free to look into other options if the treatment you're using either isn't working or seems to be working against you.

Physicians and other health-care professionals can provide much in the way of medical information, medication, and expertise. Family members and friends can provide emotional support, caring, and guidance. But you are the only one who can make the many important decisions necessary to organize your lifestyle as much as possible. These decisions may be small, but they are can be critical in determining how OA affects you and your family. To help yourself best, a whole-package approach is essential, in which you help yourself in as many ways as possible, both medically and psychologically. The rest of this book will discuss dozens of ways in which you can help yourself to improve your life with, or despite, OA.

PART TWO

Lifestyle Changes

CHAPTER THREE

Coping with Lifestyle Changes: An Introduction

So you have to make changes in some aspects of your lifestyle because of osteoarthritis? Yes, that is all part of the package. Every time you experience pain when you move, you'll be reminded that things have changed. However, changes can occur in anyone's life for any number of reasons. If you start a new job, you might have to wake up at a different time, travel to work in a new direction by a new form of transportation, or survive on a different salary. If your new job required you to move, you would have to meet a whole new group of people. If you buy a new car, you have to get used to its gadgets, as well as its quirks.

OA is an addition to your life. Although it is a condition that may never totally be cured, you can feel better, enjoy life, and do what you can. That's reasonable and achievable.

Why are lifestyle changes such an important part of dealing with OA? One of the most important goals of OA management is to relieve or reduce pain. To do this, you may need to alter your lifestyle to adapt, reduce, or eliminate those activities that may cause you pain. Changes in lifestyle can also help to prevent more damage to your joints and reduce the chance of developing deformities.

Because osteoarthritis can affect work, family life, sexuality, social activities with friends, finances, and other aspects of daily living, it is important to learn how to cope with changes in lifestyle. In some cases, these changes may be minimal. But understanding what you can do to cope with any changes that do occur can only improve your quality of life.

Your lifestyle is of your own choosing. You will automatically take many different factors into consideration when determining what your lifestyle is and what you want it to be. You can decide how full you want your days to be. You may also decide to put things off until you "feel better." But why wait? Why not try to see what you can do right now to improve the quality of your life while you're learning to live with OA?

Making Changes

One very important part of coping with OA is learning to take control over as much of your life as possible. This means taking an active part in treatment decisions and determining how all aspects of treatment can fit as comfortably as possible into your lifestyle. Keep in mind that there's a difference between taking control of your life and looking for a miracle such as your OA going away forever. Yes, this miracle would be wonderful, but hoping—and waiting—for it will not help you improve your life. In fact, it might slow down your adjustment. Ignoring your symptoms (a type of denial) can also slow down your adjustment and limit your ability to cope. So instead of looking for miracles, focus on doing the best you can to help yourself. Because the physical pain of OA can often be matched by unpleasant emotional pain, it is important to acknowledge and seek help for both types of pain.

A diagnosis of OA may seem like a totally negative thing. However, it can be viewed as positive if it serves as motivation for change or self-improvement. You see, people change and grow not only when things are going well, but also during times of adversity. By looking at your life from a different perspective, you may be able to start weeding out things that have not been good for you, and begin introducing better things. This will improve not only your own physical and emotional health, but also the well-being of those around you.

At this point, you want to change your lifestyle to make things as easy as possible for yourself. Appropriate changes can allow you to continue doing much of what you want to do without putting too much pressure on your body. In fact, as you modify your life to reduce or avoid discomfort and conserve energy, you should gradually begin to feel better. For example, try spreading out your most taxing activities. Pace yourself. If necessary, be sure to include rest periods during the course of the day so that you can recharge your batteries. These changes should help you do many of the things you want to do while taking care of your physical needs.

SET PRIORITIES

Look at yourself not as a person with unlimited strength, but as one with decreased energy. Focus on the most important things you want to do in your life, and try to spend less time on those things that don't have as much significance.

Each day, prioritize your activities so that you can spend your energy on those tasks that are most important. Make up a list of the things that need doing, and then group them into "musts," "maybes," and "possibilities." On some days, you will be able to do many of the tasks on the list; on other days, you may be able to do very few. During those times when your energy is limited, you'll be glad that you were smart enough to accomplish the most important tasks first.

Just as you must complete certain tasks each day, you should also make it a point to do some things purely for pleasure. Spend more time with people and activities that support both your physical and emotional well-being. This includes family members and others who truly care about you as a person. If it is hard to talk to your family, talk with a teacher, clergy member, or a friend whom you can trust. Spend less time—or, if you can, no time!—with people and activities that drain your strength and give you less pleasure. This will improve the overall quality of your life, better equipping you to deal with the stress of OA.

Despite all the changes you may be making to better cope with your OA, you want to maintain as much normalcy in your life as you can. Continue doing some of the things that you enjoy the most. Don't make too many changes because, if you do, you may lose track of what your life is really all about. Hobbies can help by helping you to take your mind off your condition. Find an outlet for your emotions—making or listening to music, writing, doing photography, watching movies, reading, exploring the Internet, and so on.

As you work on adapting your lifestyle, also try to gradually modify your standards, requirements, and obligations. Don't feel that you have to live up to all of your previous standards—especially if OA has diminished your strength. There is no law that says you must keep your standards at the same level throughout your entire life. Be flexible and realistic, and change as necessary to make yourself more comfortable.

Life with OA has its ups and downs. Changes may be necessary because of your emotional needs, your pain, other symptoms, and a variety of additional factors. The most efficient way to adjust is to anticipate as many of the ups and downs as possible, and ride them out as smoothly as you can.

SET GOALS

Life without goals is meaningless. Set short-term, intermediate, and long-term goals for yourself. For instance, you might choose the next book you'd like to read, find a new hobby or interest you'd like to pursue, or plan your next vacation. Then keep moving toward these goals. This will help you to put the things in your life into proper perspective.

LIVE LIFE ONE DAY AT A TIME

Live each day one at a time. Although this may seem incompatible with having goals, it's not. You can continue to live one day at a time even though you have goals in the back of your mind to give your life focus. Enjoy life as much as you can. Try to add pleasure to some of the ordinary, mundane things to which you previously gave little thought. If you go for a ride in your car, for example, instead of focusing on your destination, enjoy the process of getting there. Look at the scenery around you. Admire the beautiful things that life has to offer. At the same time, don't neglect planning for the future. You may find a treatment that provides pain relief at certain times. A positive attitude results if you address the emotional re-actions as well as the physical pain.

Getting Used to the Changes

What are some of the factors that will determine how well you'll adapt to the changes in your lifestyle? There are many. For example, what were you doing before you started experiencing OA discomfort? How satisfied were you with your work and leisure activities? How supportive were the people close to you—both family and friends? How has your condition affected you, both physically and emotionally? These and other factors will play a role in determining how you'll adjust to OA, its treatment, and the changes it necessitates. But that doesn't mean your hands will be tied. You can im-prove the way you deal with virtually every aspect of osteoarthritis.

Yes, there will be some changes in your lifestyle. But why assume that all of them have to be negative? Isn't it possible that some of them might be for the better? Maybe you were such a hard worker that you never spent enough time with your family. If you have to cut back on your work sched-ule because of OA, perhaps you'll enjoy the increased time you'll have to spend with your family. Learning to take better care of yourself will pay off in the long run. So don't convince yourself that your life is ruined just be-cause your joints are giving you a hard time! Always look at the positive in any situation. We'll be discussing how to deal with as many of the nega-tives as possible.

How About Denial?

What happens if you decide *not* to consider any possible changes in your lifestyle? This may indicate that you're trying to deny your problem. De-nial is a very common coping strategy. And believe it or not, denial can be a positive technique. How? It can help by keeping you from dwelling on problems that aren't helped by dwelling! On the other hand, denial has its negative side, too. What if denial keeps you from doing what you need to do? For example, what if you don't get enough rest, or you're too active, or, or, or . . . ? This is *destructive denial,* and it can hurt you. Hopefully, the fact that you're reading this book in the first place shows that you're not really denying inappropriately. But continue to stay on top of this.

Ingredients for Successful Coping with Lifestyle Changes

You'll be in the best shape to adapt successfully to changes in lifestyle if you:

- Understand what makes you tense.
- Know what you can and cannot do to change or avoid the symptoms and problems associated with OA.
- Pay attention to yourself—your desires and needs.
- Elicit the help of the people around you. Use relationships as a buffer. Join together with others to tackle the cause of your stress.
- Use laughter and humor to reduce stress.
- Concentrate on your strengths and accomplishments rather than dwelling on negative thoughts.
- Follow a healthy diet. Especially avoid beverages with caffeine, because too much caffeine causes nervousness, irritability, and problems with digestion and sleep.
- Get enough sleep. Allow time for rest and quiet and don't solve problems at night or when tired.
- Exercise to reduce the effects of stress by bringing blood to the muscles and the brain and stimulate production of the chemicals that give you a sense of well-being.
- Have fun in life. Have hobbies or other pursuits that you enjoy, and spend time with them.
- Realize that you need to do things for yourself, and actively think of yourself apart from pain and tiredness and the problems of this disease.

- Learn all you can about OA and seek out appropriate professional help. It is important to recognize when to ask for help—medical, emotional, spiritual—whatever it takes.
- Work on enhancing your relationship with your partner.
- Relax to reduce your experience of pain.

Keep your mind, body, and spirit in the best shape possible, so you can conquer anything that comes along.

Guidelines for Change

There are a number of things you can do to make any changes necessitated by your condition easier and less stressful. The following are some general guidelines for living with OA.

Make your house user-friendly. Reorganize rooms, work areas, and other parts of your home (and life) to maximize efficiency and convenience. Every bit of energy you conserve by making things easier for yourself around the house—including the use of appliances, structural changes, clothing modifications, and more—can be funneled into areas that will better enhance your overall lifestyle. Similarly, try to arrange your tasks so that they flow naturally and easily from one to the other. For example, try to avoid trips back and forth to different rooms of the house.

Try to plan your activities in advance, and alternate rest periods with prolonged periods of activity. For example, you might want to plan on ten minutes of rest for each hour of activity.

Limit strenuous activity and avoid excessive physical and emotional fatigue and strain. For example, try to avoid carrying things. When shopping, make use of shopping carts or bags rather than carrying items in your hands. Whatever activity you undertake, try to avoid excessive bending, straining, or reaching. Sit if you can, rather than standing. Be aware of how your body feels—how it reacts to different activities. Then act accordingly, resting as necessary. Learn your "pain threshold." If you know when you have reached the limit of how much pain you want to endure, you can slow down or stop, give your joints a rest, and not chance damaging them. The following are a number of specific tips many people with OA have found helpful:

- For activities such as reading or watching television, sit in a chair. You can strain your neck doing these activities while reclining on a bed or couch.
- Try to avoid sitting on too soft a seat. If you start feeling uncomfortable while sitting, get up and walk around.
- When you do rest, make yourself more comfortable by using support and positioning aids made of foam, visco-elastic, or some other supportive but soft material. Mattress pads, pillows, wraps, and other products provide cushioning, comfort, and support. They are also light enough to be moved around the house as necessary or to take with you when you travel.
- If you do not already own a cordless telephone, consider investing in one and keep it close to you. This will eliminate the need for rushing to answer a ringing phone.
- When driving, take frequent breaks. It's not good to sit or hold your head in one position for too long. And make sure you have "healthy" shock absorbers in your car. They can reduce the bounce and motion, and help your own personal shock absorbers feel better!
- If you anticipate that your mobility will be limited, even temporarily, obtain a temporary handicapped parking permit from your town. In most cases, you'll need a letter from your doctor saying that this is necessary. It may take time to get this permit; act now so it will be available when you need it.
- Pamper yourself a little, and learn that you don't have to do everything yourself.
- Give yourself permission to indulge in the things you enjoy.
- Accept help from others when necessary, and don't overextend yourself.
- Build on the talents and activities you can still enjoy—and there are sure to be plenty of them! Try to focus on the things that you still have, rather than what you have lost. This guideline can be applied to relationships, activities, abilities, and interests.

- Simplify your life. Work to reduce the pressures that you place on yourself by focusing on the tasks that must be done and temporarily shelving those that are less urgent.
- Be more protective of yourself. Establish and follow routines that will supply you with the proper amounts of sleep, exercise, and nutrition.
- Improve your ability to communicate. Communication problems are the main reason relationships dissolve. By learning how to best discuss important issues you will not only decrease the chance that your existing relationships will fail, but you'll also increase the likelihood of establishing new, more enjoyable ones.
- Maintain control over your life, and do as much as you can—without exhausting yourself, of course.

What's the best way to make lifestyle changes? Always remember that you are the most important ingredient in the recipe for successful adjustment. So do everything you can to help yourself. All of your efforts are sure to reap invaluable benefits in the form of greater health and happier day-to-day living.

As We Move On

Yes, you may have to make some changes in your lifestyle. But some of them will probably be for the better. Maybe you've been such a hard worker that you've never spent enough time with your family. If you have to cut back on your work schedule because of OA, perhaps you'll truly enjoy the increased time you'll be able to spend with your partner or children (or grandchildren). Certainly, learning to take better care of yourself will pay off in the long run. So as you modify your lifestyle, be sure to look for the positive. In the remaining chapters of Part II, we'll look at ways to better cope with pain, fatigue, and other effects of OA and its treatment. We'll also look at diet, exercise, and medication—in other words, at many of your lifestyle concerns. So read on, and let's get your act together!

CHAPTER FOUR

Physical Changes

Unfortunately, there may be some physical changes in your body because of OA. Although effective management may control the symptoms of OA, it will not reverse damage that has already occurred.

What can you do? Well, you won't be able to do something about all the physical changes, but many of them can be helped. So first concentrate on those things you *can* do something about. Then work on learning how to accept and live with the ones you can't change. That may seem like a tall order, but what choice do you have? After all, you're still the same person inside, aren't you?

Let's discuss two of the more common physical changes that may occur with OA—fatigue and joint problems—and how to better cope with them. (Pain has a chapter all to itself.) Is there anything you can do about these changes? Several suggestions will be offered. If you can't use them, at least you'll be learning more about the changes, and you'll become aware that you're not alone in experiencing them.

Fatigue

Do you become tired more easily? Does your bed seem to be your favorite place in the whole world? If so, you're not alone. Fatigue (yawn!) is a very common problem for individuals with OA, although it is caused more by the pain of the disease than by the disease itself. Your entire body reflects the pain you're feeling. You're more tense, you hold yourself differently, and you move differently. Whew! Exhausting! You may find that simply getting up, washing, and getting dressed makes you tired. You may be pooped for the rest of the day.

WHY DOES FATIGUE OCCUR?

Osteoarthritis can cause fatigue in a variety of ways. First, pain is very exhausting. It can drain you of energy. And pain at night may interfere with restorative sleep—you awaken already tired, and with muscles that haven't healed from the prior day's stresses. But sometimes, fatigue may be totally unrelated to OA or its treatment. You may simply be doing too much. In addition, good nutrition is critical for a healthy body. Your nutritional status, poor dietary habits, and an insufficient intake of vitamins and other nutrients can make you feel more tired than you should be.

Fatigue can also be related to your emotions. Emotions such as stress, tension, anxiety, and depression contribute to fatigue. In other words, you may be tired because of the way you feel emotionally—not so much because of physical exhaustion.

Sometimes fatigue can snowball. If you're chronically tired, you may reduce your day-to-day activities, and this may result in even more fatigue. Unless something happens to break this chain, you may find that you have less and less energy. Fatigue can also result from reducing or eliminating exercise, either because you don't want to exercise, or because pain makes it too difficult. But the less you do, the more out of shape and tired you'll become. (See Chapter 9 for more on this topic.)

Most people think of fatigue as negative, but this is not always the case. It can be positive. How? Usually, fatigue is your body's way of telling you that you need rest. If you never felt tired, you would push yourself too much! So if you become fatigued on a regular basis, discuss this with your doctor. Together, you'll be able to decide what is the most likely cause and how to eliminate it.

WHAT CAN YOU DO?

What's the best way to cope with fatigue? Rest. (How clever!) Getting a good night's sleep or taking short naps during the day are great for coping with fatigue. Other strategies for dealing with fatigue depend on its nature and cause, of course, but you should always make sure that you get the proper amount of rest so that your body can be nourished and heal.

Although rest may not make your fatigue disappear, it can certainly help. If fatigue is a message that your body is unable to do as much as you want it to do, rest is certainly an important way to gain more control. One problem, however, is that *too much rest* can lead to more fatigue! This can start a vicious cycle.

Make sure you're getting the proper amounts and types of exercise. Exercise helps to break the cycle of fatigue and deconditioning. In fact, studies suggest that walking, as well as other moderate forms of exercise, can significantly decrease fatigue. Exercise helps circulation, and better circulation clears waste products from the body. It strengthens muscles and helps injured cells to heal because they get more oxygen. Another benefit of exercise is that it helps to reduce other potential causes of fatigue like depression, anxiety, and insomnia.

Efficient planning and pacing can also reduce fatigue. Determine your exact responsibilities and schedule activities so that you're not doing too many strenuous things in a row. Make sure you intersperse rest periods with any strenuous activities you need to do. And be flexible. You can never be sure when you're going to have energy, or when you're going to feel too tired to do anything. Be ready to change course if fatigue hits you out of the blue, or if you have a sudden burst of energy!

Be willing to ask for help. Have other people accomplish some of the tasks that are lower priorities for you or that don't demand your personal attention. This will conserve your energy, allowing you to do those things that are more important.

Eating a proper diet is as critical as rest and proper pacing. Try to eat regular, well-balanced meals. Also speak to your doctor about nutritional supplementation, which ensures that you're getting the nutrients, vitamins, and minerals that are vital for a healthy body. (More information on diet appears in Chapter 8.)

Other techniques that you will learn while becoming an efficiency expert, such as reorganizing your home to make things more convenient, will also help you to do more and feel less fatigued. Don't feel as if you have to make all these changes by yourself. Professionals can give you advice that may help to improve how well you function day to day.

Finally, consider that your fatigue may be caused or worsened by emotions. Try to determine which feelings are contributing to your fatigue. (Are you depressed? Stressed? Tense? Bored? Anxious?) Then work on improving your outlook. (Chapters 12 through 19 should help you pinpoint and control any emotional problems you may be having.)

Joint Problems

Joint problems are the causes of the main physical complaints in osteoarthritis. Other than pain, stiffness (especially after resting) is a very common characteristic of OA. After awakening in the morning or after sitting or standing still for a short period of time, your body may stiffen up. Fortunately, this is usually doesn't last very long. After a brief period of loosening up, movement may become easier and less painful.

WHY DO JOINT PROBLEMS OCCUR?

As we saw in Chapter 1, osteoarthritis causes deterioration of the cartilage lining the ends of bones that form various joints. The ends of the bones may also become thicker in response to the bones grinding together, and bone spurs may develop. As a result of these factors, the space within the joint narrows. This leads to a stiffening of the affected joint. The stiffness is usually relieved by rest, and is most pronounced after periods of inactivity. Most people with OA experience the worst joint stiffness in the morning.

WHAT CAN YOU DO?

The primary treatment for joint problems involves medication and physical therapy (these will be discussed in Chapters 6 and 9, respectively). But there are other things that can be done, too. You'll want to do everything you can to protect your joints from further damage or stress. There are three basic ways to protect your joints: pacing, joint positioning, and support devices.

Pacing

Learning how to pace yourself is very important for protecting your joints. By doing too much, you put added stress on your joints, so pacing yourself, alternating periods of rest and exercise, can help to keep your joints functioning better. Whenever you are active, listen to your body. Stop doing anything that causes you pain. Include rest periods in your routine anytime you have to participate in heavy, repetitive activities.

If you're stiff, try to loosen up slowly, gradually, and gently, but recognize that it may still take a little time for your joints to become more mobile. Make sure you're taking medication at the proper times.

A warm (not hot) bath or shower may be helpful. Gentle exercises may help to loosen you up. Anticipate that you will experience a certain amount of stiffness each day. Work it out of your joints as comfortably as you can.

Joint Positioning

Learning how to position your joints most efficiently enables you to get more things done with less impact on your joints. Use larger, stronger joints to handle heavier work. Whenever you have a choice, use a larger joint rather than a smaller one. For example, your wrist is a larger joint than your knuckles. Therefore, when possible, use your wrist instead of using your fingers. In the same way, try using your shoulder instead of your elbow, and so on. Distribute your weight over several joints. For example, use two hands to lift something heavy, instead of one.

Try to extend your joints as much as possible in all activities. People with joint problems tend to keep them slightly contracted (flexed). Why? When you're in pain, a slight contraction of the joints is usually more comfortable. This is because flexing makes use of stronger muscles than extension. Although extending your joints (opening them fully) can keep joints mobile, it may be slightly less comfortable when you do so.

Try to avoid placing too much pressure against small joints of the hand (such as the back or pads of your fingers). This can put too much stress on the weakened joints to the knuckles. Use your palms instead of your fingers whenever possible.

Try not to allow joints to remain in any one position for too long. In other words, if you have to hold something—whether it's a cup, glass, book, or cards—try not to hold it in the same position for too long. Change positions as often as you reasonably can. Avoid lifting whenever you possibly can, for it is a very stressful activity.

Support Devices

There are very few things that inspire the apprehensive emotional reactions that support devices, such as wheelchairs, walkers, crutches, splints, braces, or canes, do. Why? Many people are afraid of "giving in" to their disease by using such devices. Although they know that they might be more comfortable using these devices, the fear focuses on becoming dependent on them, and worrying that, somehow, their use might contribute to a further deterioration of health. People who feel this way may offer excuses for not using devices, such as, "Using my joint is better than resting it," "If I can't do something without assistance, I'd rather not do it at all— or at least wait until I can do it without assistance," or "If I use this, it's only a matter of time until I need something that's even more advanced." But using support devices can so expand one's potential activities—for example, taking longer walks, doing more chores, suffering less pain, or going on trips—that true reasons for avoidance should be explored, especially if the devices are medically prescribed.

What exactly are the benefits of support devices? They can help those joints in the hands, ankles, feet, hips, or knees. They preserve and protect them (sounds like the U.S. Constitution!) and allow for as much functional mobility as possible. These devices may also help by spreading out the weight that would be placed on any weight-bearing joints. Use carts, such as a luggage or shopping cart, so you can roll items instead of carrying them. Use larger or longer handles on items to make them easier to hold or use. Take advantage of the many household devices that can help you by minimizing movements that involve twisting, turning, or gripping. The numbers of different types of support devices—and their uses—are virtually unlimited. (For more information about support devices, see Chapter 10.)

A Physical Finale

So there are physical changes as a result of OA. This chapter has included only the two most common ones. You may not be thrilled with them. But once again, what's the alternative? You do want to learn how to cope with OA and the changes that result from it. That's why you're reading this book, right?

CHAPTER FIVE

Pain

Ouch! (Just getting you ready for this chapter!) Is osteoarthritis painful? Are you kidding?! Most individuals with OA believe that the pain is the hardest thing to deal with. But the good news is that treatment for OA is designed to improve the quality of your life and decrease your discomfort.

What is pain? Pain is a type of sensation picked up by nerve endings and transmitted to the brain. This message is very important. Why? Pain is a signal from your body telling you that you're having trouble in a particular part. In OA, it can tell you that a joint is injured or that you're using a damaged joint too much. It also signals you to "slow down" to prevent additional damage. As a result, pain can be an important diagnostic tool. Only *you* know the intensity of your pain. Pain suggests that you rest the injured areas of your body so that your tissues can be repaired. It can help you to determine the nature or severity of an illness or injury. Only after these messages travel from the site of irritation to the brain do we feel pain.

What can you do about your discomfort? How can you cope with it? The best way to cope with pain is to get rid of it! To do this, it's first necessary to identify the cause of the pain.

What Causes Pain?

Although it's still not completely understood what causes the pain of OA, it is generally believed that the pain results when the nerves in the joint become irritated. The pain of OA may be caused by physical changes in the joint, or by pressure on the nerves by osteophytes. Inflammation can contribute to pain as well.

Earlier in the development of OA, only movement may trigger pain. Eventually, however, pain may increase to the point where it might occur during rest periods as well.

When Does Pain Occur?

The stiffness and pain of osteoarthritis are intermittent—they do not necessarily occur constantly. Pain typically occurs during or following activity. For the lower extremities, pain may occur as a result of weight bearing even if there is no movement. Pain often occurs early in the morning upon awakening, after rest periods, or during damp or wet weather.

Many factors may contribute to your pain—not only physical factors, but also psychological and environmental ones. Although pain may initially be physical, emotions can quickly worsen, or exacerbate, the pain. So pain may result from stress, fatigue, or depression.

Stress causes you to tense your muscles. It may make it more difficult for you to relax, and can increase the degree of pain that you're experiencing. If you're fatigued, you may feel more pain because your tissues and joints aren't getting the rest they need to repair themselves. Depression may cause you to feel more pain too, because your OA is frequently on your mind.

When you're in pain, this may increase the degree to which you experience stress, fatigue, or depression. This can lead to more pain, creating a vicious cycle.

Treatment for Pain

Once you're aware of what's causing your pain, treatment can attempt to eliminate the cause. But what if you can't do anything about the underlying source of the pain? At least you can try to get some relief from it.

How can you start to deal with pain? First, be aware of your pain. One of the most important steps you can take is to use a diary and record when you feel the pain, where you feel it, how often it occurs, how long it lasts, and how intense it is. This will help you decide if the pain is something you can handle yourself, or if it's serious enough to be brought to your doctor's attention. Remember: If in doubt, check it out.

Next, provide your doctor or health-care professional with an accurate description of the pain. Describe exactly when and where you feel the pain. Indicate how long you've had it and how long it usually lasts. Note whether the sensation is steady, sharp, throbbing, or dull. Also describe the intensity of the pain—whether it is mild, moderate, or severe. You'll also want to be able to distinguish between pain and stiffness, and be familiar with the pattern of your pain. You can rate your pain using a pain scale that will help your doctor to understand what you are experiencing and provide the most appropriate treatment.

There are four traditional categories of therapy for pain control: chemical (using medication), surgical, physical (physical therapy), and psychological. In general, all four therapies work by either eliminating the trigger to the pain or interrupting the transmission of pain messages before the brain receives and interprets them.

Medical treatment for pain generally involves medication. This can effectively control a lot of problems. For example, acetaminophen (Tylenol) and aspirin have been effective in controlling minor pain. But sometimes discomfort will continue, despite the use of medication. (The next chapter will go into much more detail on medication.) In extreme cases, surgery may be helpful in treating the cause of the pain. But not all conditions lend themselves to surgical treatment. (Surgery will be covered in Chapter 7.) So it may be necessary for you to learn other techniques for dealing with pain.

Other than medicine and surgery, what are other ways of trying to obtain pain relief? Physical techniques (such as using TENS units, heat, cold, hydrotherapy, acupuncture, and massage) and a proper balance of rest and exercise (to be discussed in Chapter 9) can be used, as can psychological techniques such as imagery, biofeedback, yoga, hypnosis, and relaxation. (More about all of these later in this chapter.) Last, but not least, it is very important to maintain a positive attitude.

You can learn how to employ techniques for controlling pain from physicians, physical therapists, occupational therapists, and mental-health professionals such as psychologists who may specialize in certain pain control techniques. Or you may want to read some of the many books on pain that can be found in bookstores and libraries. (See For Further Reading in the back of this book for some suggestions.) Many techniques for pain control can be applied at home, although in some cases treatment in specialized clinics or centers may achieve greater success.

Despite the effectiveness of the pain control techniques mentioned in this chapter, it is important to consult your physician to make sure that any or all of the techniques you are interested in are appropriate for you. Make sure that anything you're thinking of using will not be dangerous for you, considering your condition.

Now let's go on to discuss some of these pain-control techniques.

TENS UNITS

TENS stands for *t*ranscutaneous *e*lectrical *n*erve *s*timulation. TENS units have been gaining in popularity to help control pain. Each unit is a little box about the size of a pack of cigarettes. It contains a generator that has wire leads with electrodes at the ends of them. The unit may have anywhere from two to forty electrode wire leads. To use one, you attach a little gel to the electrodes, then place the electrodes on your skin, on or near the area to be treated. When you turn on the unit, a low level of electricity flows into the area from the TENS unit. This stimulates the nerve fibers and blocks the transmission of pain messages to the brain. Shocking, right? Don't worry. You probably won't even feel anything, or you may experience a mild tingling sensation.

One of the problems with TENS units is that their effectiveness seems to decrease as time goes by. The effectiveness of the TENS units also seems to be related to your diligence, the knowledge of your therapist, and the appropriate placing of electrodes.

If you want to get a TENS unit, you usually need a prescription from your physician. A nurse or physical therapist can then teach you how to place the electrodes to provide you with maximum pain relief. But it's probably a good idea to rent a machine before buying one to see if it works for you.

HEAT AND COLD

Both heat and cold treatments can be beneficial in the temporary relief of OA pain and stiffness. However, neither has an effect on the disease itself. If you're going to use either heat or cold, be careful! You can hurt yourself if you misuse it. And neither should be used if you have poor circulation or have any other medical condition that would be exacerbated or damaged by them.

Some people seem to benefit more from heat; others seem to benefit more from cold. This may vary within you as well, depending upon the stage of your disease. There may be times when they work best in combination. At other times, different joints may benefit from different approaches.

Heat

Heat can be a very beneficial way of relaxing and soothing your muscles to relieve soreness and pain. This is called thermotherapy. It may be the oldest form of pain reliever, or analgesic, in the world.

When heat is applied to a selected area of the body, it increases the temperature in that area. There are two good reasons for doing this. First, it increases blood circulation to the area. And second, it increases the metabolic rate.

If you are using heat, you should feel comfortably warmed and relaxed. By relaxing tight muscles, you can increase the mobility of your joint. (This is one reason why using heat before exercise can be helpful.) Usually, positive effects from heat can be felt in about twenty minutes, give or take a few minutes. However, trial and error is necessary to find out what's best for you.

IS HEAT ALWAYS HELPFUL?

Heat may not always be appropriate. If an affected joint is treated with heat, it may aggravate symptoms in this joint. For example, there may be increased swelling or damage. Heat may be harder to tolerate for the very young or very old.

If you are going to use heat, be careful about the intensity and duration of its use. Too much heat for too long a period of time (more than twenty minutes) is not advisable. Don't assume that if a little bit of heat is good, a lot of heat can be better. This is a good way to get burned!

WAYS TO APPLY HEAT

The methods of applying heat may be divided into two categories: moist heat and dry heat. Examples of moist heat include using hot towels or specially designed hot packs (such as Hydrocollator pads), hydrotherapy, or water baths. Hydrotherapy can be used for both hot and cold applications. Dry heat can be applied using hot water bottles, electric heating pads, microwaveable gel pads, or heaters.

Is there a difference between the effectiveness of moist heat and dry heat? Not very much. Both can be effective as long as the frequency, duration of treatment, and intensity are controlled. However, some ways of applying heat may be more effective for large areas of your body, while others may be more effective for small areas. Let's discuss some specific heat treatment techniques.

Hot packs. One way to apply moist heat is by using warm, damp towels or hot packs such as Hydrocollator pads. Hot packs can be very helpful in relieving pain and reducing inflammation. A hot pack is usually made up of a canvas sack that contains a heat-retaining silica gel. (That's why it may also be called a gel pack.) It is heated in hot water, wrapped in terry cloth, and applied to the painful area for about twenty minutes. The silica gel contained in the hot pack can retain heat for a long period of time. Or you can make your own hot compresses of towels. This involves soaking a towel in hot water, then wringing it out and applying it to the painful area.

If you use hot packs or hot compresses, be careful to avoid burns! In general, a good way to avoid burns and retain heat for longer periods of time is to use plastic sheets or dry towels wrapped around the hot compress.

Warm baths. A warm bath in the morning is a great idea. Not only can it be very helpful in reducing the stiffness and pain you'll feel upon awakening, but you'll get clean in the bargain! Hot showers also can reduce stiffness. Many muscles can be relaxed at the same time. Usually baths or showers should last no longer than twenty minutes. Why? They may make you tired, even in that short period of time.

Paraffin wax treatments. Paraffin wax treatments, using melted wax, are a good way to apply heat to the hands. (Make sure you initially use these treatments under the supervision of your doctor or physical therapist.) Usually, the painful area is dipped in melted wax ten to twelve times. This forms a very thin, glove-like layer that covers the area, coats it, and keeps it warm for a fairly long period of time. Once the wax is in place, the joints must remain still or else the wax will crack. After fifteen to forty-five minutes, the wax is peeled off. Because of the close adhesion of the wax to the body, is not a good idea to use paraffin treatments on any body part that has an open wound. It's also important to be very careful while heating the wax, to avoid fire hazards.

Heating pads. Electric heating pads can be helpful but should not be used for long periods of time. They should be placed on top of the painful area. It's not a good idea to lie on a heating pad or fall asleep with one on. Heating pads are usually safest at low settings.

An electric blanket or mattress pad may also be helpful. Not only do they provide warmth, which can be soothing to your joints, but they also mean that you will require fewer blankets in cold weather. So what, you say? Well, if you need fewer blankets, you won't have to bear the weight of a large number of blankets on your already weakened joints! Get it?

Obviously, if you use any electrical appliances, use them carefully. And be sure to take any precautions necessary to avoid burns.

Cold

Although there are many benefits to using heat treatments, some people and situations respond better to cold treatment. Cold treatments, also known as cryotherapy, can help the painful joints of OA. How? Cold has a numbing effect on nerve endings in the affected areas so you won't feel so much pain. It also decreases the activity of the body cells.

One common method of cold treatment involves soaking a cloth or towel in ice water, wringing it out, and applying it to the painful area. Gel packs, which can be obtained from pharmacies and medical supply stores, are an excellent means of applying cold and, because of their pliable consistency, are often more comfortable than ice packs. These gel packs are kept in the freezer, removed for use, and then refrozen. Of course, if you don't have a gel pack, ice cubes or a frozen wet cloth placed in a plastic bag can be just as effective. Some people have even found it effective to apply a bag of frozen peas to a painful site! As with hot compresses, be sure to wrap these applications in a towel before holding it against the skin.

Like heat, ice should be used only for short periods of time—not longer than ten to twenty minutes each time. Treatments can be repeated as necessary or desired, but let your skin return to normal temperature before using it again. And, of course, make sure you follow professional recommendations regarding how to use any of these techniques or procedures.

Some people don't like cold treatments, saying that they're only good for polar bears. Others, however, find that they provide greater pain relief than heat treatments. Some people derive benefit from heat and cold applied alternately. This can increase blood flow to the area, which can have the effect of removing body chemicals involved in generating the pain from the area, while bringing in substances that can help in repair and pain reduction.

Contrast Baths

Contrast baths may be helpful in relieving pain and swelling for some individuals. If you use them, you will be contrasting hot and cold water treatments. The most common procedure used for contrast baths is to soak the extremities for three minutes in hot water (at approximately 110°F) and followed immediately by one minute in cold water (at approximately 65°F). This procedure can be repeated several times, as needed.

HYDROTHERAPY

Hydrotherapy, or water baths, may be a very helpful way to get your joints more mobile, as well as to promote relaxation, improve deep breathing, increase circulation, reduce swelling of the extremities, and improve coordination. Hydrotherapy can also be helpful as a heat technique.

But hydrotherapy can cause fatigue, so it should not be done for long periods of time. And you should have somebody there with you, if possible, in case you do become drowsy.

POOL EXERCISE PROGRAMS

Pool exercise programs, also called aquatics by the Arthritis Foundation, can be very beneficial for your OA. (They can also be helpful if you don't have the disease!) You can exercise many parts of your body in the water. Exercising in pools is safe and much less hard on the joints than doing the same exercises out of the water. It can also be more enjoyable! You're more likely to build up the strength of your muscles and range of motion in your joints when you're in the water. It's possible to do much more in water than out of the water. Movements are easier in the water because weight is relieved by its buoyancy. You'll be able to more easily move joints that are weakened and painful. The warmth tends to reduce the pain and spasms of muscles.

There are many centers that have specific aquatics exercise programs for individuals with arthritis. Check with your local chapter of the Arthritis Foundation for further details. (See the Resource Groups section in this book.)

ACUPUNCTURE/ACUPRESSURE

Acupuncture and acupressure are examples of traditional Chinese medicine, and may be effective for some people in treating arthritis. Acupuncture is administered using hair-thin needles inserted into specific body points. Acupressure is a form of massage that applies finger pressure on acupuncture points. Practitioners often use a combination of these methods. Both are used to stimulate or sedate the body's flow of vital energy along channels, or meridians. This helps disperse and dissolve any kind of blockages that may be in those meridians. (According to traditional Chinese medicine, illness is a consequence of imbalance or blockage of *qi*, or vital energy, in the body.) Make sure you look for a licensed acupuncturist in your area.

MASSAGE THERAPY

Massage may be the most ancient and natural pain reliever of them all. Massage offers many physical benefits for people with OA, such as decreasing muscle tension and stiffness, lowering blood pressure, stimulating circulation, relieving pain, and restoring movement in the joints. Therapeutic massage is deep and relaxing, and gives your body a chance to rest and sleep (a time for repair and healing). Some people believe that healing energy is locked in the muscles and that massage can release energy blockages and help eliminate chronic pain..

ALLEVIATING PAIN PSYCHOLOGICALLY

Is pain purely physiological? Rarely. It's usually a combination of physiological and psychological factors. What does this mean? Although your joints may be hurting, it's your *mind* that determines just how much it hurts.

Angela was moving exceptionally slowly, primarily because she had a lot of pain in her knees. The pain overwhelmed her every time she tried to move faster. Even when she was doing something she enjoyed, her movements were restricted. Suddenly, she heard her 66-year-old husband cry out. Without thinking about her joint pain, she went flying across the room to see what had happened. How could her pain have been purely physical? Yes, Angela had been in pain, but her mind had probably magnified it. When she had realized that her husband might be in trouble, her pain had temporarily taken on secondary importance.

What does all this mean? If medication or other medical interventions don't help alleviate your pain, you can still relieve some (if not all) of it by working on your mind's awareness of it. Read on to find out how you can do this.

Relaxation Techniques

You know that tension can actually increase your pain. So it makes sense that relaxation—the opposite of tension—can help you reduce your overall level of pain. As an added benefit, using relaxation techniques may increase your general sense of well-being and help you deal better with the stress of many day-to-day problems—not just those related to OA.

There are a number of different types of relaxation procedures, including progressive relaxation, meditation, autogenics, deep breathing, and a method called the quick release. Let's look briefly at each of these techniques.

Progressive Relaxation

Progressive relaxation is based on the premise that when you experience anything stressful, the body responds with muscle tension—which, of course, can increase pain. In this procedure, which is usually performed for fifteen to twenty minutes once or twice daily, you sequentially tense and then relax the different muscle groups in your body, one group at a time. If you wish to learn more about this popular and effective technique, don't hesitate to consult books at your local library or speak to a professional.

Meditation

Meditation is a valuable tool for stress reduction. It really is a name for any activity that keeps the attention pleasantly anchored in the present moment. When the mind is calm and focused in the present, it is neither reacting to memories from the past nor being preoccupied with plans for the future, two major sources of stress. Meditation can allow you to achieve a deep level of relaxation in a short period of time. During meditation, you focus your mind, uncritically, on one object, sound, activity, or experience, and "clear out" any extraneous thoughts. Depending on the type of meditation you choose to use, this technique usually works best when taught by a professional or learned from a reliable book or videotape.

AUTOGENICS

Autogenics is a systematic program that helps you train your body and mind to respond to your own verbal commands to relax. With this procedure, which can be used for short periods of time and repeated as frequently as needed, you give yourself verbal suggestions of heaviness, warmth, and calmness. Again, a book on relaxation techniques or a qualified professional can guide you in the use of this procedure.

DEEP BREATHING

Many people find that deep breathing can significantly increase their relaxation and, as a result, decrease their pain. Deep breathing can be used in a number of different ways. One simple deep-breathing exercise is the following: First, assume a comfortable position on your bed or on the floor. Then put one hand on your abdomen and the other on your chest. Inhale slowly and deeply through your nose, so that the hand on your abdomen moves higher. Hold your breath as long as you're comfortable doing so; then exhale slowly through your mouth, making a peaceful "whooshing" sound. Feel the hand on your abdomen sink slowly, and allow a growing feeling of relaxation to deepen inside you. Repeat this sequence for five to ten minutes. Then give yourself a few minutes to become aware of your surroundings before getting up. Practice this technique at least twice a day, extending its length if you wish.

QUICK RELEASE

Another simple but effective relaxation technique is the quick release. To do this, close your eyes, take a deep breath, and hold it as you tighten the muscles in every part of your body that you can think of—your fists, arms, legs, stomach, neck, buttocks, and so on. Continue to hold your breath and to keep your muscles tense for about six seconds. Then let your breath out in a "whoosh," and allow the tension to drain out of your muscles. Let your body go limp. Keep your eyes closed, and breathe rhythmically and comfortably for about twenty seconds. Repeat this tension-relaxation cycle three times. By the end of the third repetition, you'll probably feel a lot more relaxed. Keep on practicing this technique, as continuous practice will condition your body to respond quickly and completely.

In addition to those described above, you may find other relaxation techniques that are helpful. Remember that your ability to increase relaxation and decrease pain by means of the mind-body connection is limited only by your imagination. Don't overlook this valuable way of improving your sense of well-being.

Imagery

Imagery is the process of conjuring up mental pictures or scenes in order to harness your body's energy. These images, which can occur spontaneously or can be guided in particular directions, are multisensory—that is, you can see, hear, feel, smell, or taste them in your own mind. By using positive mental images, you may be able to more effectively cope with and reduce pain. Guided imagery often results in a positive physical response that reduces stress, slows the heart rate, and stimulates the immune system. The technique can be used to control headaches, hypertension, depression, and pain. Sometimes used alone, imagery can also be used in combination with prescribed medical treatment.

How can you use imagery to control the pain of OA? Get into a relaxed position in a comfortable chair or in bed. The lights should be dimmed, and outside sounds or noises should be minimized. Try to avoid interruptions. Breathe smoothly and rhythmically, allowing your body to release tension and relax. Then imagine a scene of your own choosing, trying to make the image as vivid and real as possible. This scene can be used therapeutically to help you feel better.

Anita was suffering from a sharp pain in her knees. She was instructed to relax and then develop an image of what this pain looked like. She imagined it as a very sharp knife being jabbed into her knees. (Alternatively, she might have pictured her knees being hit by a hammer or having dozens of pins stuck into them. Whatever the imagery, it should be as vivid and detailed as possible.) Anita was then instructed to reverse what was happening in the image: She imagined the knife slowly being removed from the knees, and a soothing cream being applied. Finally, the knife was completely out. She was then able to relax and her discomfort was eliminated.

There are other images you can use to reduce joint pain. For example, you could imagine cool air being blown across the affected area, oil or a soothing lotion being gently massaged into the affected joint, or being surrounded by warm water in a bathtub. Imagery is restricted only by your creativity, and can be used anywhere. (Have you ever taken a bath on a bus?!) Two good books on the subject are *In the Mind's Eye* by Arnold Lazarus and *Visualization for Change* by Patrick Fanning. See if your public library or local bookstore has them. (More information about these, and other useful books is found in the For Further Reading section of this book.)

Imagery is also a key component in hypnosis. You might choose to use hypnosis, since it can be helpful in pain control.

Biofeedback

Biofeedback uses the techniques of relaxation and imagery in conjunction with modern technology to teach you how to change and control your body's vital functions. Simple electronic devices measure your body's physiological responses and give feedback in the form of sounds or images, letting you know what's going on inside your body. In fact, biofeedback provides moment-by-moment information about the effect that your imagery and relaxation techniques are having on your physiological responses. What do I mean by physiological responses? Skin temperature, the electrical conductivity of the skin, muscle tension, heart rate, brain wave activity are all physiological responses that can be measured for the purposes of using biofeedback.

How, exactly, can biofeedback help you control pain? Electrodes connected to the biofeedback unit are taped or otherwise attached to your skin. Then you use meditation, relaxation, visualization, or some other technique to bring about the desired response. These electrodes monitor your body's response and transmit the information they pick up to the biofeedback unit in the form of electrical impulses. The unit then translates this feedback into sounds, lights, or pictures that you can hear or observe. Using this information, you can experiment and find the types of imagery and other relaxation techniques that will allow you to best control your pain.

Glenda was experiencing a lot of joint pain in her shoulder, so her physician suggested she try biofeedback. A machine measuring muscle tension was attached to her shoulder in much the same way that electrodes from an electrocardiogram (EKG) machine are connected. (Don't worry. There is no pain, and you won't get jolted!) As Glenda attempted to relax, the machine gave her instant feedback as to whether she was really relaxing, and also how well she was doing. As she became aware of her lessening tension, Glenda learned what mental images worked best for her. Eventually, she was able to use the imagery on her own, without the machine, to help her relax and control some of her pain.

Not much research has been done specifically on the effects of biofeedback for people with arthritis. However, research has indicated that biofeedback can teach people how to relax and help them to control pain, warm their hands, and get their muscles to work effectively. This may be helpful for individuals with OA.

Certified biofeedback professionals can be found throughout the country. Good resources for names of local practitioners include your physician, local hospital or clinic, and the Association for Applied Psychophysiology and Biofeedback. (See Resource Groups in this book.)

Psychological Coping Strategies

There are other factors that can contribute to the intensity (even the very existence) of your pain, including your emotional state, the attention you pay to your pain, and the way the rest of your body feels. Obviously, as you pinpoint which of these factors does play a role, you can begin improving the way you cope with pain.

Where do you start? You want to do everything you can to decrease fear, stress, tension, and other negative emotional factors. Anything you can do to relieve anxiety and tension (including psychotherapy, if necessary) should help you to cope better with any pain.

How do you reduce the amount of attention focused on your pain? Of course, the more time you have to think about it, the worse it will seem. So try to divert your attention. Develop other interests that require concentration. You can always come up with pleasant thoughts or activities that will distract you from painful thoughts. A very helpful activity might be to get involved with a support group for people living with pain. One such organization is the National Chronic Pain Outreach Association. (See Resource Groups in this book.) They have many chapters throughout the country, and more are always forming. It can be great to know that you're not alone in trying to cope with pain. Who knows? You may even get some great ideas that will help to reduce the pain you have to live with!

An Unagonizing Conclusion

Whether your pain comes from OA, your treatment, or something else, don't throw in the heating pad! Realize that the pain need not last forever. A lot can be done, both medically and psychologically, to help deal with it.

CHAPTER SIX

Medication

Some people welcome drugs as a powerful way to control problems in the body. Others are afraid of their power and of eventually becoming dependent on them. Still others resent the presence of any artificial substances in their bodies. Where do your feelings fit in? Regardless of what your attitudes are toward using medication, your physician has probably made it clear that you don't have much choice in the matter. One of the components of a comprehensive treatment program for OA is taking medication. This can help you to live a more comfortable life. How? The main reason medication is prescribed for OA is to reduce pain. It can help you feel better, and keep your joints moving! Regardless of how important your medication is, you must remember to take it properly. Otherwise it can be very dangerous.

Choosing the Appropriate Medication

How does a doctor determine which medication should be used? In prescribing a drug program, your physician will take into consideration your overall condition, as well as the symptoms you are experiencing, other treatment being used, any other drugs you may be taking for other conditions, your age, and your overall health, among other factors. If, in the past, you have shown sensitivities to any drugs, you should certainly let your doctor know—even if you think this information is already part of your medical record. The more facts your doctor has on hand, the better chance he or she will have of finding the right treatment for you.

Although doctors consider many factors before prescribing medication, your doctor cannot predict exactly how a given medication will affect you. So in many cases, a certain amount of trial and error is necessary to determine the best medicine and the optimum dosage for you. You may need to try different kinds of medication over long periods of time in order to arrive at the combination that can best help your condition. This can be frustrating, but keep in mind that the right drug—or combination of drugs—may greatly increase your comfort level. So try to be patient!

How and When to Take Your Medication

Whenever your doctor prescribes a medication, be sure you understand exactly what the medication is supposed to do, and how and when it should be taken. For example, certain medications should be taken only after meals, while others must be taken on an empty stomach. In still other cases, specific foods must be avoided during drug therapy.

Each person has different needs as far as dosage and frequency are concerned. Even if someone you know has the same symptoms that are troubling you and is taking the same medication, his or her dosage may not necessarily be appropriate for you. And once you start taking the medication, your dosage may have to be adjusted based on any side effects you're experiencing and how well the medication is managing your symptoms.

Once you begin taking the prescribed dose of a medication, don't start taking more (or less) on your own. Because of the chemical natures of drugs and the way they act in your body, it is extremely important that you follow your doctor's instructions when taking the drugs prescribed for you.

Medications can be administered in a variety of ways. They can be taken in pill or liquid form; by injection; through rectal suppository; or by intravenous (IV) drip. In some cases, a pain pump (also called a medication pump) may be recommended. This is a device that can be either implanted in or worn next to your body. It allows you to administer prescribed doses of painkillers to yourself as needed.

You probably want to take as little medication as possible. Very few physicians will keep you on high doses of any medication unless they feel it's absolutely essential. Still, if you're taking a substantial amount of any drug and question the need for such a dose, don't be afraid to ask your doctor about it. A good doctor should be willing and able to explain your program. If you're feeling good and would like to try reducing your dosage—or to stop taking the drug altogether—by all means, speak to your doctor. Together you will be able to plan a schedule for reducing your dosage and, if possible, ending treatment.

Before taking any medication, make sure to ask your doctor or pharmacist the following questions:

- What is the name of the medication?
- How and when do I take it?
- What is it supposed to do for me?
- What side effects may occur with this drug?
- What do I do if I develop any of these side effects?
- How long should it take for the drug to show results?
- When should I contact the doctor if I haven't noticed any results?
- Are there any medications, foods, activities, or other things that I should avoid while taking this drug?

They Might Not Get Along!

Never take any medications other than those prescribed for you without first checking with your doctor. If you need to take a number of different pills, it's important to avoid playing with your dosage, playing with the times you take them, or moving around the number of pills you take at a particular time. Follow your doctor's prescription as carefully as possible.

If you see physicians other than those who are handling your OA, be aware that they may prescribe medications that absolutely should not be taken with some osteoarthritis medications. Thus, the advantage of having one primary physician in charge of your care is obvious. Any other doctor you see can then consult with your primary physician to make sure that the treatment strategies will work together. Because certain medications are chemically incompatible, you should never mix drugs without first knowing that the combination is safe. Don't take the chance. Check it out. And always make sure that each of the doctors you're working with knows about all the medications you're taking.

There is always the chance that certain drugs, including over-the-counter ones, may not be appropriate in your OA treatment program. You've heard this a lot already, but it's important: Check with your doctor! Ask questions, learn, and help yourself. Consult with your physician before taking even the most innocent over-the-counter drug. You never know when you might have a bad reaction.

Side Effects

Very likely, you are concerned about the possible side effects of any prescribed medication. Side effects, as you know, are the less-than-pleasant effects a drug may have on your body. Nausea, dry mouth, increased or reduced appetite, sleep disorders—these are all possible side effects of certain drugs. In fact, side effects are probably one of the biggest concerns about medication.

Because medication causes chemical changes within the body, side effects may occur whenever a drug is taken. And, unfortunately, the more powerful the drug, the more potent its side effects may be. If the side effects you experience are slight, you will probably want to ignore them—especially if the medication you're taking is having the desired effect. Even if the side effects are disturbing, you may want to continue the medication if its benefits outweigh any discomforts you're experiencing. However, if side effects are having a particularly harsh impact on you, you should inform your physician, and the two of you should weigh the disadvantages against the advantages. In fact, you should report any side effects to your doctor so that he or she can determine if the drug therapy should be continued, changed, or ended. Be aware, however, that the "side effects" of *not* following prescribed treatments may include pain, stiffness, or joint damage, among other problems.

With any drug, it is important to find the lowest effective dose. This is one way to maximize the productivity of the medication and, hopefully, minimize any side effects. Taking the medication exactly the way it's been prescribed for you may also minimize side effects. Again, if there are any problems, call your doctor!

Getting Down to Specifics

Let's talk about some of the medication taken for OA. The goal? You want to learn all about any medicine you have to take as part of your life, so that you can cope with the changes. Fortunately, many people with OA need only one type of medication. But because medications work differently for different people, there are a lot of different kinds out there!

The primary reason to use medication in the treatment of OA is to reduce pain. In the past, nonsteroidal anti-inflammatory drugs (NSAIDs) were the treatment of choice for the pain of OA. But recently, the American College of Rheumatology (ACR) developed new OA treatment guidelines. They define the three major categories of medications to reduce the symptoms of osteoarthritis as the following:

- Aspirin-free pain relievers.
- Nonsteroidal anti-inflammatory drugs (NSAIDs).
- Corticosteroids.

Let's look at each of these three categories, some of the newer drugs being used to treat OA, and other drugs that may also be helpful in your overall treatment program.

ASPIRIN-FREE PAIN RELIEVERS

In drug treatment for osteoarthritis, pain relief is usually all that is necessary. Therefore, the first-line drug therapy for OA is the use of an aspirin-free pain reliever. The primary drug in this category is acetaminophen (better known by the brand name Tylenol). It is used for temporary relief of mild to moderate pain. Not only does it not contain aspirin, it does not commonly irritate the stomach. However, it does not reduce swelling and inflammation. The ACR selected acetaminophen as the first-line drug of choice because of its effectiveness, safety, and cost. The ACR guidelines point out that several research studies have proven acetaminophen to be comparable in effect to the NSAIDs in treating OA pain. It can usually be taken safely except by people who drink alcohol to excess.

Other than Tylenol, examples of drugs containing acetaminophen are Aspirin-Free Anacin, Aspirin-Free Excedrin, or Panadol.

NONSTEROIDAL ANTI-INFLAMMATORY DRUGS (NSAIDS)

Nonsteroidal anti-inflammatory drugs (NSAIDs)—so named, cleverly, because they reduce inflammation but don't contain steroids—are currently considered the second-line treatment for OA. These drugs work to relieve pain and reduce inflammation. So if acetaminophen doesn't ease pain, NSAIDs can be the next step in treatment.

NSAIDs reduce your ability to feel pain. They also block the production of substances called prostaglandins, chemicals that help trigger and prolong the inflammatory process. You will experience inflammation in those joints where prostaglandins have been released. These prostaglandins seem to increase the pain you experience because they sensitize nerve endings. NSAIDs interfere with the production of prostaglandins and, as such, block pain and reduce inflammation.

Some NSAIDs are available over the counter, whereas others must be prescribed by your doctor.

Side Effects

NSAIDS can cause a variety of side effects. Stomach upset is common. You may experience nausea, heartburn, or indigestion. Vomiting may occur. Usually, taking NSAIDs with food, milk, an antacid, or a drug specifically prescribed to deal with such symptoms can prevent or alleviate some of these discomforts. Sometimes these side effects can be avoided by using special types of coated pills known as enteric-coated pills. Another side effect from high doses of NSAIDs is tinnitus, a ringing or buzzing in the ears. Dizziness, slight losses of hearing, or slight changes in vision may also result from continued use of these drugs. However, when the dosage is lowered or the drug is stopped, these side effects almost always go away. Make sure to let your doctor know if you experience any of them.

More Serious Problems

There are some people who should not take NSAIDs. Some asthma sufferers may not be able to tolerate them. NSAIDs can cause bleeding and, on rare occasions, may even lead to severe gastric hemorrhaging from ulcers. People with gastrointestinal problems should always use great caution if told to take NSAIDs. People who are using other types of medication, such as blood thinners, should also be advised to avoid them. In addition, NSAIDs may affect the kidneys and worsen high blood pressure; they may cause fluid retention and cause congestive heart failure.

People who are allergic to NSAIDs must avoid them. (People who are allergic to aspirin *can* be allergic to NSAIDs. Tell your doctor.) There is a difference between allergies and side effects. If you are allergic to NSAIDs, you must eliminate any such drugs from your treatment program; however, if you are experiencing side effects, you may still be able to use the NSAID if you adjust the dosage or take other measures. Symptoms that suggest an allergic reaction include a rash, a runny nose, and wheezing. On the other hand, symptoms such as ringing in the ears, headache, nausea, abdominal pain, and stomach upset are more likely to be side effects.

Why is it so important that you recognize the possible side effects of NSAIDs? If you are taking these drugs for a long period of time, it is possible you will develop some of these side effects. If this occurs, talk to your doctor. You may be advised to reduce the dosage slightly, in order to determine exactly what the best dosage is for you. Changing to a different brand may also reduce side effects.

Don't give up on NSAIDs too quickly. However, if you experience any of the allergic symptoms mentioned above, these can be more serious. You should then stop taking the drug and notify your physician immediately.

Examples of NSAIDs

There are many different types of NSAIDs. The main differences between them are primarily biochemical in nature, and are beyond the scope of the book. NSAIDs available without a prescription include aspirin (found in Anacin, Bayer aspirin, Bufferin, Ecotrin, and other products); ibuprofen (Advil, Motrin IB, Nuprin, and others); ketoprofen (Orudis KT, Actron), and naproxen sodium (Aleve).

Examples of some of the more common prescription NSAIDs include indomethacin (Indocin), naproxen (Naprosyn), piroxicam (Feldene), and tometin (Tolectin), as well as higher-dose formulations of ibuprofen (Motrin) and ketoprofen (Orudis). Newer NSAIDs are coming out all the time.

OTHER PAINKILLERS

Narcotic analgesics are much more powerful drugs than nonnarcotic pain relievers. These drugs work by changing your perception of pain and creating a heightened sense of well-being. Unfortunately, they can also be habit-forming and frequently cause side effects, including nausea, vomiting, or drowsiness.

Examples of these analgesics include hydrocodone (in Vicodin and other products), meperidine (Demerol), oxycodone (Percodan, Percocet, and others), and propoxyphene (Darvon, Darvocet).

REGARDING PAINKILLERS . . .

In general, there are two main disadvantages to the use of any of the painkillers we've discussed. First, your body may become used to painkillers fairly quickly. As a result, they become less effective after a period of time and you need to take more of them to produce the same effect. This phenomenon is known as *tolerance.* You may need to continuously increase your dose so that it keeps working, and, with some drugs, this can lead to addiction. Your addiction may be psychological as well as physiological. And second, as we've discussed, painkillers can have significant side effects, and increasing the dosage increases the likelihood of them. These side effects can add to the problems that come with your condition.

CORTICOSTEROIDS

If your arthritis does not respond to prescription NSAIDs, doctors may prescribe corticosteroids for you. Corticosteroids (called *steroids* for short) are the third-line drug treatment for OA. They have been shown to be effective in treating a number of arthritic diseases. Corticosteroids are similar to a natural body hormone called cortisone that is produced by the cortex of the adrenal glands. Today, all corticosteroids used in the treatment of disease are produced synthetically and are available only by prescription.

Corticosteroids are very powerful, effective anti-inflammatory drugs. They can quickly reduce pain, inflammation, allergic reactions, asthma attacks, and colitis attacks. But although they can relieve inflammatory symptoms very effectively, they do not correct the underlying cause of any disease. Most physicians advise against the use of oral steroids for OA because of the potential for severe side effects. Also, steroids should not be used for extended periods of time, and OA is a chronic condition.

Since steroids are usually not part of treatment for OA, what's the point of mentioning them? Well, there are times when injecting steroids directly into a joint affected by OA can give quick relief. For example, if your knee joint is so painful that you are unable to comply with other aspects of your treatment program (such as exercise), or if you cannot walk at all, local injections of steroids may help to improve your mobility and reduce pain. Painful joints may become free of pain for fairly long periods of time. This will allow you to exercise as well as to participate more comfortably in your daily activities. Hopefully, exercising during this period of respite will strengthen your muscles and loosen your joints sufficiently so that you can eventually continue your treatment program without steroids.

There is another advantage to injecting steroids directly into a joint—you won't experience any of the usual side effects seen with oral steroids. But there are a few problems with steroid injections, such as the possibility of joint infection where the needle enters the body, or the risk of repeated injections causing cartilage damage or destruction. They should be used only several times a year *at most* because of the risk of weakening bone and cartilage.

If affected joints are weak or if cartilage destruction is severe, steroid injection is not recommended. And if a number of joints are affected by OA, it may be unwise, or even impossible, to inject each joint.

OTHER TYPES OF MEDICATIONS

Much research is focusing on the development of new medications to fight OA. Some of the promising new arrivals on the scene are COX-2 inhibitors, hyaluronate, and tramadol. Topical medications may also be useful for pain relief. In some cases, antianxiety medications and antidepressants may be prescribed for people with OA. Let us look briefly at each of these kinds of medications.

COX-2 Inhibitors

COX-2 inhibitors have been getting much attention as effective pain relievers that cause fewer side effects than do NSAIDs. COX is actually an abbreviation for cyclooxygenase, an enzyme. The body produces two kinds of cyclooxygenase, designated COX-1 and COX-2. All currently available anti-inflammatories inhibit both COX-1 and COX-2. Why is this a problem? Without going into too much detail, COX-2 is part of the inflammatory response that results in pain and inflammation. On the other hand, COX-1 is basically a good enzyme. It helps to protect the stomach and regulate blood pressure in the kidneys. As a result, when you take a standard anti-inflammatory drug that inhibits both COX-1 and COX-2, you might experience side effects such as stomach bleeding and high blood pressure, particularly in the kidneys. So scientists have been working to develop drugs that selectively block the effects of COX-2 but leave COX-1 (the good one) alone. That is basically what's been developed in two drugs, celecoxib (Celebrex) and refecoxib (Vioxx). These drugs are known as COX-2 inhibitors. They work in the same way as other anti-inflammatory drugs but, happily, studies have documented that they are safer for the gastrointestinal tract. The incidence of gastric ulceration and gastrointestinal bleeding were reported to be significantly lower with these drugs than with conventional NSAIDs.

Tramadol

Tramadol (Ultram) is another analgesic that has been approved by the U.S. Food and Drug Administration (FDA) for the treatment of OA pain. Tramadol is neither an NSAID nor a narcotic analgesic, and is reported to have fewer side effects than either of these two types of drugs. The most common side effects are nausea, dizziness, constipation, and headaches. Monoamine oxidase (MAO) inhibitors, drugs sometimes prescribed for depression, should not be used at the same time as tramadol.

Hyaluronate

Hyaluronate is a purified form of hyaluronic acid, a chemical that is a normal component of healthy joint fluid. In people with OA, the quality and amount of hyaluronate often is deficient. It can be injected directly into a joint in the form of sodium hyaluronate (Hyalgan) or hylan G-F 20 (Synvisc) to act as a joint lubricant. Injections of this fluid can be beneficial for some people with OA.

Topicals

Topical medications, those that can be rubbed directly onto a sore area, are another option for treating OA pain. These topicals are available in cream, gel, lotion, and spray form. Most of them contain substances called *counterirritants* that make the skin feel hot, cold, or itchy.

Topicals should not come in contact with wounds or sores, or with the eyes, mouth, or other mucous membranes. They should not be used along with NSAIDs, and they should be applied sparingly. Do not use counterirritants more frequently than the manufacturer's directions suggest. Wear gloves while rubbing them on, and wash your hands immediately after using them. (Of course, if you're using them *on* your hands, don't wash your hands right away!)

Because some topical products contain salicylates, you shouldn't use them if you are sensitive to aspirin. If you have asthma or nasal polyps, use topicals with caution (in some cases, aspirin can trigger asthma or induce nasal polyps, although this is less likely to occur with topical formulas). Don't use a heating pad while using a counterirritant; this can lead to burning of the skin. Watch for developing skin irritation, nausea, vomiting, or ringing in the ears, and discontinue use of the topical immediately if you experience any of these side effects.

Examples of over-the-counter topicals include creams and lotions such as Absorbine Arthritis Strength, Absorbine Jr., Aspercreme, Bengay, Heet, Mineral Ice, Myoflex cream, and Sportscreme.

Capsaicin, a compound derived from hot peppers, is available in a topical cream (Zostrix). It has been shown to be more effective than traditional analgesic creams. It can be used with oral medications, while most topicals cannot (other topical creams have medications in them that should not be used with NSAIDs).

ANTIANXIETY DRUGS AND ANTIDEPRESSANTS

There are two other categories of medication that may be part of the treatment for OA: antianxiety drugs and antidepressants. There are several drugs in each category. Although they may generally work in the same way, there are at least minor differences between them. So if one prescribed medication has an unpleasant side effect, another drug from the same category may be able to give you the same benefits without the side effect. And if the prescribed drug is not making you feel better, another medication may do the trick. Your doctor will work with you to find the medication that works best with your particular body chemistry and that is compatible with any drugs already being used in your treatment.

Antianxiety Medications

There are times that people with OA can be affected by anxiety. Many people have been able to reduce their anxiety through nonpharmacological methods—relaxation techniques, exercise, and other forms of stress management. (Anxiety will be covered in detail in Chapter 15.) But if medication seems to be the answer for you—and especially if your anxiety is intense, or leads to panic attacks—there are three subcategories that may be helpful.

The first group of antianxiety medications are the *benzodiazepines*. There are many drugs in this group, represented by alprazolam (Xanax), chlordiazepoxide (Librium), and diazepam (Valium). The latter two, though effective for controlling anxiety, are not considered as effective for panic attacks. Benzodiazepines have few side effects, but can be habit-forming.

The second subcategory of drugs primarily used in the treatment of anxiety are the tricyclic antidepressants. These medications were actually among the earliest ones found to be effective in dealing with panic, but are now used less often, since more effective medications have been found. The drugs in this category include imipramine (Tofranil) and desipramine (Norpramin).

The third subcategory of antianxiety drugs are the monoamine oxidase (MAO) inhibitors. Some doctors consider these to be the most effective for panic control. However, of the three groups, this one requires the greatest care in following dosage schedules and other precautions in order to minimize side effects. For example, if you're taking a MAO inhibitor, it is important to avoid taking antihistamines or decongestants, as the drugs might be incompatible and cause further problems. Also, foods with high concentrations of the compounds tyramine or dopamine—aged cheeses, beer, and wine, for instance—should be avoided, as the combination can lead to episodes of dangerously high blood pressure. Examples of drugs in this subcategory are phenelzine (Nardil) and tranylcypromine (Parnate).

When using antianxiety medications, keep in mind that even when they are effective, they are really only blocking the anxiety or panic attacks. It is still important to deal with the triggers of the anxiety, and to implement any changes necessary to resolve the problems that led to the anxiety in the first place.

Antidepressants

Unfortunately, depression can be a common problem for people with OA. Nonmedical coping techniques can often successfully deal with depression. (These are discussed in Chapter 14.) If problems persist, though, a number of different antidepressants may be helpful. Examples include tricyclic antidepressants such as desipramine and imipramine; and MAO inhibitors such as phenelzine and tranylcypromine sulfate. These medications work in different ways, and can cause different side effects. Other antidepressants include amitriptyline (Elavil), doxepin (Sinequan), fluoxetine (Prozac), maprotiline (Ludiomil), nefazodone (Serzone), nortriptyline (Pamelor), paroxetine (Paxil), sertraline (Zoloft), trazodone (Desyrel), and venlafaxine (Effexor).

Work with Your Pharmacist

Many people rely solely on their doctors for information about prescribed medications. If this is true of you, you're overlooking a wonderful information resource: your pharmacist. Pharmacists know a great deal about drug interactions, about which foods should be avoided when taking certain medications, and about other possible problems. So it can be helpful to develop a good working relationship with your local pharmacist, and to go to that same person for all your medications.

Besides being a good source of information about drug actions, your pharmacist may be able to help you reduce costs. How? He or she may be able to suggest a less expensive brand name or generic drug. While there may be nothing wrong with the substitute drug, in some cases certain formulations may work better than others. So always be sure to consult your physician before changing brands. (Depending on how your doctor fills out a prescription, your pharmacist may *have* to contact him or her before substituting a brand other than the one specified.) A good relationship with a well-informed, helpful pharmacist can benefit you in more ways than one.

Additional Medication 'Minders

Once you have begun taking a medication, let your physician know if the drug is having the desired effect. Any significant changes in your health, whether good or bad, should be reported to your physician. This will enable your doctor to make an informed decision about whether your current drug program should be continued or changed.

If you find that you're having trouble remembering to take your medication—or if you're sometimes unsure if you've already taken a dose—find ways to keep track of your medication schedule. For instance, you might prepare a daily chart that lists each dose separately and allows you to check off each one as you take it. You might also purchase a multicompartment pill box, which can store a week's worth of drugs, divided into appropriate days and times. Some even sound an alarm when the time comes for you to pop your pill!

As previously mentioned, certain drugs are chemically incompatible with one another, or may be incompatible with other aspects of your treatment. For this reason, it is essential that you put together a list of all the medications you are taking, and that you keep this list in your wallet. You will then be able to show the list to your doctor, your pharmacist, or anyone else who needs to know what you're taking.

A Final Prescription

Medications are only one part, although an essential part, of your overall treatment program for OA. This chapter couldn't, of course, include every medication used by people with OA. And new drugs are developed all the time. Always discuss your medication with your physician. If you hear of new drugs on the market, ask about them. They may not necessarily be better for you than your existing medication, but you won't know unless you ask.

Hopefully, the information presented in this chapter has given you a good idea of what you must know in order to use medication as safely and effectively as possible. There's a lot to learn, but the more you understand about your medications, the more likely you are to benefit from them. So if your doctor prescribes something new, ask about it. Not only will you probably feel a lot better as a result of taking the medication, but you'll also know *why* you're feeling better!

CHAPTER SEVEN

Surgery

Not too many people cherish the thought of "going under the knife." In the past, surgery as an OA treatment technique was rarely considered except as a last resort. But in recent years, because of advances in surgical technology, surgery has been considered more often in the treatment of OA. When the amount of pain or the limitation in activities because of OA becomes overwhelming, surgery may be considered. So let's discuss surgery, and the way it can affect your lifestyle.

When can surgery be helpful? If other approaches (such as medication, rest, and physical therapy) fail to alleviate pain or to reduce disability or deformity, surgery may be considered as an alternative. However, most arthritis experts recommend trying all other treatments before considering surgery. If your OA is so severe that it causes constant excruciating pain or significantly limits your mobility, then surgery may be necessary. In such cases, it can be very effective in helping you return to a more satisfactory, active life. It can relieve pain and restore comfort and mobility to joints affected by OA. It can also be useful in correcting serious deformities.

Surgery for OA is usually elective. Although you may feel you need it because of pain or disability, it's usually not something that is done on an emergency basis.

Why Surgery?

If joint cartilage is worn away as a result of OA, the joints may become painful, stiff, weak, or unstable. If this damage becomes severe, then excruciating pain, loss of function, and deformity may result. Weight-bearing joints may be affected to the point that you have great difficulty walking. If OA seriously affects your upper extremities, you may find that you're barely able to perform even the simplest activities of daily living.

If your OA affects only one joint or a few joints, surgery may return you to a virtually pain-free existence. If more joints are affected, surgery won't cure OA, but at least it can significantly relieve many of the problems that come with it. Surgical procedures can currently be used on individuals of virtually any age, although your age and overall physical condition will be evaluated to decide if surgery is desirable for you.

There are some reasons that surgery may not be appropriate for everyone. Surgery can be painful and expensive, and can require a long recovery period. It also keeps you away from certain activities that you normally enjoy. You may argue, though, that your condition before surgery prevented you from doing these things anyway. If you have certain medical problems, such as a heart condition or lung disease, surgery may be contraindicated, since it may pose a higher risk.

There are a number of questions you should ask your doctor before deciding on surgery. They include:

- Can current treatment continue to result in improvement so that surgery would not be necessary?
- What are the risks involved in the proposed surgery?
- What are the risks of not having, or delaying, the surgery?
- How likely is it that any of the risks may occur?
- What kind of improvement can result from the surgery?
- How long will the recovery period take?
- What is involved in rehabilitation following surgery?
- What limitations will be in effect after the surgery, and how long will they last?

Types of Surgery

There are several types of surgery performed for OA. They can be used to repair bone deformities, fuse joints, rebuild joints, or even replace your own joint with an artificial joint. In determining what type of surgery is to be done, the orthopedic surgeon must consider several factors, including your condition, which joints are affected, the degree to which your joints have been affected, and your age and lifestyle.

ARTHROPLASTY

An increasingly common surgical procedure for osteoarthritis is arthroplasty. This refers to any surgical procedure that restructures a joint. There are two types of arthroplasty, involving reshaping or replacing damaged joints.

Reshaping Damaged Joints

In this type of arthroplasty, parts of a damaged joint surface are removed. A surgical reformation, or shaping, can help to rebuild damaged joints. In this procedure, the ends of the bone where cartilage has worn away are resurfaced or relined. This eliminates the problem of bone or ligament damage due to cartilage erosion. Arthroplasty may actually create a false joint, where only some of the bone in the joint is removed or the bones are realigned.

This type of surgery is less frequently done these days. Why? Although a partial restoration may restore some function, it may not eliminate pain. Weight-bearing joints may still prove to be unstable. The trend today seems to be away from these partial resolutions to the problem and toward total joint replacement.

Joint Replacement

The second type of arthroplasty is joint replacement. In joint replacement surgery, the old joint is removed and replaced by an artificial one (a prosthesis), usually constructed of plastic and metal. This type of surgery is commonly done for the hip, knee, and shoulder.

The most common joint replacement surgery is for the hip. The hip joint is the largest joint in the body. It's also one of the most important weight-bearing joints. A problem in this joint can certainly affect you. For example, the hip joint can become rigid and unusable. The pain may make any kind of movement almost impossible.

Several thousand total hip replacements are done each year. It has gotten to the point where hip replacements are considered almost routine surgery—successful more than 95 percent of the time.

Total joint replacement for the hip is the most frequently performed (and successful) arthroplasty operation. This procedure aims to resurface both the acetabulum (the cup) and the femoral head (the ball) surfaces of the hip joint. Knee joint replacement surgeries are also quite successful. Replacement of certain other joints is becoming more successful; research and experimentation continue on surgery that can replace joints in the wrists, ankles, elbows, feet, and toes.

DEBRIDEMENT

A relatively minor procedure to remove bone spurs or other bone fragments in the joint is debridement. This procedure also removes unhealthy, worn-out cartilage from the joint. Although this procedure can be very effective and can do a great job of reducing (if not eliminating) pain, there is one significant problem with it: The results from this procedure are usually not permanent. Eventually, it may have to be repeated.

ARTHROSCOPY

Arthroscopy is a surgical procedure that makes use of an arthroscope (a small periscope-type instrument) to look into the joint. The arthroscope, which is a little bit wider than a drinking straw, enables the surgeon to see practically everything that's inside the joint. The arthroscope can be useful in diagnosing problems within a joint. It can also be used for debridement purposes, in which bits of torn bone or cartilage can be shaved or removed. Arthroscopy is most commonly used on the knee, but can also be used on the hip and shoulder.

ARTHRODESIS

Another procedure used is called arthrodesis, or surgical fusion. Two bones may be fused together to stabilize and strengthen a weak joint. Although the bones in this joint will no longer be able to move (because the fusion freezes them rigidly in place), the purpose of the procedure is for the joint to be able to support weight more easily and without pain.

Surgical fusion may be used, for example, at the joint at the base of the thumb. This can help to restore at least some degree of mobility to the hand—mobility that may have been lost due to pain and restrictions. Arthrodesis may also be done on the spine if, for example, damage from OA affects the vertebrae in the neck.

OSTEOTOMY

The osteotomy is a procedure that attempts to correct a deformity in a joint. In this operation, one of the two bones in a joint is cut and reset in a better alignment. Why is this done? If the cartilage on one bone is worn away more than the cartilage on the other, the result is a bad bone alignment in the joint. Osteotomy aligns the bones in a better position.

RESECTION

A resection is a surgical procedure in which part or all of a bone is removed. This is usually done in situations in which the removal of the bone or joint will not significantly affect mobility. Resection procedures are often done on the metatarsal joints in the feet if OA makes it too painful or difficult to walk. Another use of resection is on the end of the ulna bone in the wrist, to help reduce pain and deformity of that joint.

Getting Ready for Surgery

The prospect of any kind of surgery can be frightening. The more you know about the surgery itself, the anesthesia, and your postoperative recovery period, the less nervous you will be. After all, if you know that something you are experiencing after surgery is normal, you won't have to worry that something has gone wrong. A good, caring physician will openly discuss all of your concerns with you.

What Happens After Surgery?

After surgery, it's time for rehabilitation. Your program will include rest, physical therapy, and gradually increasing amounts of activity. You will need plenty of rest. You will also need time to get used to assistive devices, such as crutches, canes, or splints, that will support the surgically repaired or replaced joints during this phase. You will probably learn special exercises to help you regain strength and mobility in the affected joint. (By the way, exercising before surgery is a good idea, because it can make the after-surgery rehabilitation more productive and comfortable.) But be careful. You don't want to take a chance of damaging the joint that has just been repaired! In all probability, it will be at least a few weeks before you can resume your usual routine. You may want to make arrangements to have someone help out at home for a while following surgery.

A Surgical Conclusion

Surgery can result in an abrupt, positive change in your condition. Hopefully this change will be permanent, but even if it is temporary, there are some important things to think about.

Although surgery can potentially relieve pain and restore a good degree of mobility, this doesn't mean that you'll be able to get involved in very strenuous physical activities! And although you may be able to do more than you did prior to surgery, there still may be differences between what you can do with artificial joints and what you were able to do with the healthy joints you had before developing OA.

Ask your primary physician for recommendations regarding who should perform the surgery. For example, you'll probably want an orthopedic surgeon for joint replacement surgery. And if surgery is being done on your hand, you'll probably want a specialist in hand surgery. Your surgeon should be someone you feel comfortable with and who also has extensive experience in exactly what type of surgery you need.

Discuss what's involved in the operation and what kind of rehabilitation will follow with your doctor. Find out what you will need to know before, during, and after the procedure. Feel free to ask questions. Remember: Preparation for surgery makes the outcome better (and easier)!

Get a second opinion before agreeing to any type of surgery. This is always important before deciding whether surgery is the treatment for you.

If you are leaning away from surgery because you know someone who underwent an operation with a less than successful outcome, make sure you properly balance this information with the positive results obtained by other people who have had the same surgery.

Prepare yourself for extensive rehabilitation after surgery. You will probably work with a physical therapist, who will prepare a plan that will help you get back in the swing of things. In almost all cases, successful surgery depends not only on the surgery itself, but on the diligence with which you participate in rehabilitation *following* the surgery.

In considering any kind of surgery, ask yourself (and the doctor) a very simple question: "Will the surgery make a big difference in my quality of life?" If so, fine. That's the reason to consider it. But it's important to know as much as you can about surgery in order to make the right decision.

CHAPTER EIGHT

Diet and Nutrition

Food, glorious food! Do you like to eat? It's one of the great pleasures of life. But are you eating more and enjoying it less? Research has shown that OA, as well as its treatment and changes in lifestyle, may affect your eating habits and, accordingly, your weight. Therefore, it makes sense for people with OA to try to control their eating patterns and eat as healthy a diet as possible.

You might have questions about whether your diet will have to change because of your OA. Or maybe friends and family members have told you that you should change the way you eat.

Is there a particular diet that is most appropriate for OA? Most experts think not. Of course, it's important that your diet be nutritionally sound and well-balanced. Why is nutrition so important, and what exactly is a good diet? A proper diet ensures that we consume all of the necessary vitamins, minerals, and supplements. In addition, eating a varied diet that emphasizes low-fat, high-fiber foods is important in your quest to maintain a healthy weight (or to lose weight, if you need to).

Let's look at the role that diet plays if you have OA, and about what you can do to maximize your health in this area.

Why Is Nutrition So Important?

Nutrition is the process of eating appropriate amounts of nutrients and us-ing them to meet energy needs, to accomplish body-sustaining healing, and to satisfy maintenance requirements. Improving your nutrition is a powerful way to create health. The human body is very complex, but it can heal itself of many disorders if you provide it with proper nourishment and care. If you do not give your body the proper nutrients, you can actually impair its normal functions and cause yourself harm. Here are just some of the benefits a sound diet may provide for the person with OA:

- A body that is well-nourished is stronger than a poorly nourished one. So proper nourishment enables the body to better fight disease, aids healing, and promotes well-being.
- Good nutrition provides good energy. Everybody needs fuel to ener-gize the body. And because of the potential energy-zapping effects of OA pain, proper diet is even more important.
- A good diet actually helps people respond better to OA treatment, and makes them more resistant to treatment side effects.
- A balanced diet increases the speed at which body tissues heal themselves.
- Without proper nutrition, the body's stores of protein, fat, vitamins, minerals, and other nutrients may be depleted in unhealthy ways. A good diet ensures continuing healthy stores of these nutrients.
- A sound diet limits fat, an important part of any program to lose weight.
- A sound diet includes vitamins A, C, B_6, and the minerals copper and zinc, which are required by the body for the manufacture of col-lagen and normal cartilage.

Dietary Recommendations

Perhaps it's best to begin our discussion by looking briefly at the United States Department of Agriculture's (USDA's) most current dietary recommendations. If your last acquaintance with nutrition included the "four basic food groups," which emphasized the importance of meat, poultry, and dairy, the new guidelines may prove startling. Basing their recommendations on current research, the USDA now recommends a complex-carbohydrate-based, low-fat, high-fiber diet. Whole grains, fruits, and vegetables are the basics of a good diet. Of lesser importance are dairy products, meat, poultry, and fish. Fats, oils, and sweets should be used only sparingly.

Certainly, the USDA guidelines make good sense for anyone. But let's take a closer look at some specific dietary recommendations for the person who's learning to cope with OA.

EAT A LOW-FAT DIET

Following a low fat diet has many benefits, such as reducing the risk of developing heart disease, breast cancer, and many other disorders. How, exactly, can you reduce the fat in your diet? Limit your consumption of red meat to about once every ten days, and eat only lean cuts. Any dairy products that you consume should be nonfat (lactose-free if necessary). And, as much as possible, eliminate saturated oils and fats, including butter, margarine, lard, and vegetable oils. When oils can't be totally avoided, use only small amounts of monounsaturated oils, such as canola and olive oil, or peanut or safflower oil, which are polyunsaturated. Get to know the good fats—such as omega-6 fatty acids (found in nuts, wheat germ, primrose oil, and borage oil), and omega-3 oils (found in fish such as salmon and mackerel). These fatty acids are believed to inhibit prostaglandin production and may be helpful in reducing inflammation and pain.

Finally, determine which foods make you feel drained of energy or bloated, or have some other unpleasant effects. Then eliminate them from your diet or, at the very least, limit the amount you eat. The foods most commonly found to have such effects include cow's milk and other dairy products, food preservatives and artificial colors, wheat, chocolate, eggs, citrus fruits, and foods containing salicylates (such as apples, cherries, grapes, peaches, eggplant, broccoli, tea, and coffee).

EAT A HIGH-FIBER DIET

Some studies focus on the theory that high-fiber diets are more healthy than low-fiber ones. How does fiber contribute to health? Fiber—the part of plant materials that our body does not digest—binds with bile acids, cholesterol, carcinogens, and other harmful substances and sweeps them through the digestive tract and out of the body. In other words, fiber is good for removing certain toxins from the body.

Because the refining process removes much of the natural fiber from our foods, the average diet lacks sufficient amounts of this important substance. Fortunately, it's easy—and delicious—to add more fiber to your diet every day. High-fiber cereals are one of the best sources. Also good are brown rice, whole-grain breads and pasta, bran, most fresh fruit, dried prunes, nuts, seeds, beans, unbuttered popcorn, and lentils. Raw vegetables and Brussels sprouts, broccoli, kale, and cabbage are also fiber-rich.

EAT A DIET HIGH IN ANTIOXIDANTS

There is a group of vitamins, minerals, and enzymes called antioxidants that help to protect the body from the formation of free radicals. Free radicals are atoms or groups of atoms that can cause damage to cells, impairing the immune system, and, many experts believe, lead or contribute to aging, infections, and various degenerative diseases. Antioxidants defuse free radicals, thus helping to preserve the cells' DNA, the genetic material necessary for healthy cell reproduction. The body itself produces some antioxidants, but there are also a number of nutrients that act as antioxidants, including vitamin A, beta-carotene, vitamins C and E, and the mineral selenium.

You should make sure to eat sufficient quantities of foods containing antioxidants, such as sprouted grains and fresh fruits and vegetables. Active vitamin A is found only in animal sources, such as cod liver oil, beef, and chicken. However, beta-carotene, which the body can use to produce vitamin A, is found in green and yellow-orange vegetables and fruits, including acorn and butternut squash, apricots, cantaloupe, carrots, chicory, dandelion greens, kale, kohlrabi, spinach, sweet potatoes, and turnip greens. Some of the foods highest in vitamin C are broccoli, Brussels sprouts, kale, turnip greens, parsley, sweet peppers, cabbage, cauliflower, and spinach. Vitamin E is found in such vegetable oils as corn, soybean, and safflower oil, and in whole grains, dark green leafy vegetables, nuts, and legumes. Selenium is found mostly in seafood and whole grains.

One final note: When adding fruits and vegetables to your diet, be sure to get the freshest produce possible, as it will have the highest levels of nutrients. If possible, eat the vegetables raw, as heat can destroy nutrients. When cooking vegetables, steam or microwave them briefly to preserve as much of the nutrient content as possible.

VITAMINS, MINERALS, HERBS, AND NATURAL FOOD SUPPLEMENTS

Vitamins are organic compounds that are essential to life. They help regulate the metabolism and assist the biochemical processes that release energy from digested food. Every living cell depends on minerals for proper function and structure. Minerals are inorganic compounds needed to properly compose body fluids, form blood and bone, maintain healthy nerve function, and regulate muscle tone. Both vitamins and minerals function as coenzymes, substances that work with enzymes to enable the body to function. Many herbs and natural food supplements contain powerful ingredients that, if used correctly, can help heal the body. Because vitamins, minerals, herbs, and natural food supplements are vital to good nutrition, it stands to reason that you can benefit from a number of these if you have OA.

Let's discuss vitamins and minerals first. The vitamin-B complex is particularly important. The B vitamins (as well as vitamin E and vitamin C) help to reduce the severity of internal inflammation and inhibit prostaglandin production. Taking a multivitamin supplement or individual doses of these vitamins can be helpful, even if you do follow a healthy diet. Minerals such as iron, calcium, magnesium, and zinc are also important. If you are taking medication that contributes to loss of bone density, you should ask your doctor about taking a formulation containing calcium, magnesium, and vitamin D. You should also ask about minerals, such as magnesium and zinc, that may help to reduce inflammation and pain.

What about taking herbs if you have OA? Herbal remedies have become increasingly popular in recent years, and have found their way onto the shelves of ordinary drugstores and supermarkets. Certain herbs, used in conjunction with diet, can promote health and well-being for people with OA. Some people with OA have benefited from using herbs such as yucca leaf tincture, devil's claw, and alfalfa leaf extract. In addition, some people have reported improvement in OA by using glucosamine sulfate and chondroitin sulfate (more about these supplements later).

Remember, some physicians are not knowledgeable about vitamins, minerals, herbs, and dietary supplements that may help with OA symptoms. Some people prefer to find a practitioner who specializes in these areas. Be sure to keep your physician informed if you decide to use any of these alternative therapies.

AVOID HARMFUL NONFOODS

In addition to some of the foods you may be eating, a number of "nonfoods"—additives, pesticides, hormones and steroids, alcohol, caffeine, and tobacco—can be damaging to your health. Let's take a brief look at each of these and why they should be eliminated from your diet.

Artificial Additives

Believe it or not, the average American diet includes 5,000 or more artificial additives used to maintain freshness and to preserve the attractive look or taste of food. While some of these additives are considered safe, others have not yet undergone sufficient studies to determine their safety. For example, monosodium glutamate (MSG) and aspartame (NutraSweet) are used without warnings, but have been known to cause a wide range of problems, including gastrointestinal upset and diarrhea. Cyclamate and saccharine are examples of additives once deemed safe but later banned or allowed to be used only if accompanied by warnings.

What can you do to eliminate all—or, at least, many—of these chemicals from your diet? Obviously, additives are most common in processed foods—canned, frozen, and prepackaged products. Avoid these foods whenever you can. Instead, eat whole foods that are as close as possible to their natural state. When you do buy prepared items, choose those that have been made without additives. In addition, don't eat smoked foods (such as bacon or luncheon meats), which contain some of the most harmful processing chemicals used.

Pesticides, Steroids, Hormones

Like additives, residues of the pesticides used by farmers to control weeds and pests are abundant in your diet. These chemicals are found in meat, poultry, fish, dairy products, vegetables, fruits, coffee—virtually all of your foods. Many pesticides are banned in the United States, but reach us through produce grown in other countries.

How can you avoid these harmful additives? Well, unless you eat only organic food that has been grown in pesticide-free soil, you consume these potentially harmful substances every day. To reduce your exposure, scrub or peel all fruits and vegetables, particularly those that are waxed. You can also clean produce with nontoxic rinsing preparations, available in health food stores. If possible, buy organically grown foods, and avoid imported produce.

Animals raised for human consumption are often fed steroids and hormones to induce growth. To reduce their effect, buy meats that are certified drug-free and eat less meat, eggs, and dairy products (something you should be doing anyway!). Finally, be aware that a diet high in fiber and antioxidants can help eliminate pesticides and other harmful substances from your body.

Alcohol

Excessive alcohol consumption is *not* recommended for people with OA. For example, if you are taking medications that may lead to loss of bone density, you should avoid alcohol because it can add to this loss. Alcohol is also incompatible with many medications, such as aspirin and NSAIDs, commonly used for pain. If you have problems sleeping, avoid alcohol in the evening and before bed. While you may think a nightcap will help you get to sleep, in fact alcohol disrupts normal sleep patterns and results in poorer-quality sleep. In addition, alcohol is known to be so damaging to the immune system that some consider it a strong immunosuppressive drug.

Is it necessary to avoid all alcohol? There's no simple answer to this question. However, it does seem wise to keep your consumption to a minimum. Many experts believe that one drink a day is a safe amount. Less is better. After all, you want to do all you can to make your body strong and healthy.

Caffeine

Like alcohol, caffeine—found in coffee, tea, cola, chocolate, and other foods—can contribute to loss of bone density and should be avoided by people with OA. And it stands to reason that you should cut out caffeine if you have sleep problems.

Again, if you want to do everything possible to strengthen yourself, it makes sense to significantly reduce or eliminate consumption of products that contain this chemical. If you wish to drink coffee, make sure it has been naturally decaffeinated using what is known as the Swiss or water process. And what should take the place of your coffee, tea, and other caffeine-containing beverages? Your best bets are skim milk, soymilk, mineral water, unsweetened fruit juices, and vegetable juices. Besides eliminating harmful caffeine, most of these drinks take a further step toward improving your health by supplying valuable nutrients.

Tobacco

Finally, let's talk about tobacco. Everyone knows that tobacco and secondhand smoke have been implicated in several life-threatening conditions, including cancer, heart disease, and stroke. Smoking also causes great damage to the immune system and it, too, contributes to loss of bone density. Chewing tobacco and snuff have been found to be just as harmful as cigars and cigarettes. Tobacco is also a stimulant and causes sleep problems in many individuals.

In the case of tobacco, the best course of action is clear. By avoiding all tobacco—including secondhand smoke—you will strengthen your body against not only OA but also a number of other diseases.

GLUCOSAMINE AND CHONDROITIN

Glucosamine sulfate and chondroitin sulfate are nutritional supplements—available without prescription at health food stores—that have been the subject of numerous books and articles. Proponents say that they can stop, and even reverse, the effects of OA—and without side effects, to boot. Let's look briefly at these supplements and what is known about them.

Glucosamine is a natural substance found in the body and made up of glucose (simple sugar) and an amino acid, glutamine. It is a primary ingredient of proteoglycans and glycosaminoglycans, water-retaining molecules that build, lubricate, and nourish cartilage, keeping it smooth, moist, and flexible. (See page 5.) Glucosamine also serves to stimulate cells called chondrocytes, which help in the production of more of these two molecules.

Chondroitin, another natural substance, works to attract fluid in the proteoglycan molecules (nourishing the cartilage and enabling the fluid to act as a spongy shock absorber), and inhibits certain enzymes that otherwise destroy cartilage.

The theory is that sufficient amounts of these natural substances are produced by the body and supplied by diet when we're young. But aging reduces the body's ability to repair cartilage, and the body then requires more of these substances than it produces or takes in through diet.

Each of these supplements can be used independently to produce good results. But using them together is believed to increase their effectiveness in promoting the formation of cartilage, repairing cartilage and joint tissue, and preventing cartilage breakdown. The popularity of these supplements, therefore, is due to the belief that they may play a role in halting—and reversing—the damage caused by OA.

Ongoing studies are focusing on the benefits of these supplements for people with OA. The best advice at present is to discuss their use with your physician and nutritionist.

Losing Weight

Weight control is very important for people with OA. Why? Added weight can put more pressure on joints such as the knees and hips (which bear much of the body's weight), worsening pain and increasing stiffness and inflammation. If you are overweight, you will certainly want to lose weight.

Why are you overweight? Don't blame this on your OA! Your weight may increase or decrease and your appetite may change, but this fluctuation probably has nothing to do with your medical condition. Maybe your weight is fluctuating because of weekend binges! Maybe you've gone to some food orgies! Maybe you've been more sedentary and taken to snacking more than usual. Maybe emotional crises have caused you to overeat. Whatever the reasons, stay on top of this.

There are practically as many programs to lose weight as there are people needing to lose weight. Some of them are very healthy and can be incorporated into your routine (with the approval of your health-care team). Others, however, should be avoided because they may simply not be healthy. No matter what program you use, it is essential to work on modifying your eating routine. And make sure that your health-care team approves any program that you are considering.

Some people just need to maintain their weight by adjusting their caloric intake and including moderate exercise in their routines. Others need to lose weight, and want to reduce calories and increase exercise.

You may choose to work with a dietitian to set up weight-loss goals and an eating plan that will best help you to achieve your goals, especially if you have a lot of weight to lose. But any plan should take time. In most cases, a strict weight-loss program is not necessary (and sometimes is more difficult to follow for the duration). A well-balanced, nutritional, commonsense approach to eating is the best way to lose weight. Don't try to lose weight too quickly. You want to develop an eating plan that you can comfortably live with for the rest of your life.

Getting Started

Now you know why a good diet is an important part of your overall treatment program. So it's time to get started making the changes necessary to create the healthiest diet possible! Here are a number of suggestions that may be helpful.

- Keep a food diary by writing down everything you eat. This will give you a realistic look at your present diet, and will suggest ways in which you can make improvements.
- Drink plenty of fluids—at least eight glasses of fluids each day.
- Decrease the fat in your diet by limiting your consumption of meat, cooking oil, butter, and margarine, and increasing your consumption of fresh fruits and vegetables and whole grains.
- Decrease your consumption of dairy foods, and make sure that the dairy foods you do eat are nonfat.
- Eat all foods in a form as close as possible to their natural state. This will maximize their vitamin, mineral, and fiber content, and minimize additives.
- Do what you can to avoid harmful nonfoods—additives, pesticides, alcohol, caffeine (found in coffee, tea, sodas, and chocolate, for example), and tobacco. While you may not be able to avoid all these substances all the time, by cutting down on them as much as possible you'll be doing a great deal to improve your overall health.
- Minimize empty calories. Cookies, potato chips, candy, and the like have little or no nutritional value, and may keep you from eating vitamin- and fiber-rich foods. In addition, many of these foods are laden with fat.
- To help ensure an adequate intake of vitamins and minerals, consider including vitamin and mineral supplements in your dietary program. Speak to your doctor about which supplements would be best for you.
- Eat regularly. If digestion occurs on a regular and frequent basis, your blood sugar level will be kept from fluctuating wildly, and you'll

enjoy greater energy and fewer mood swings. Frequent, smaller meals may be the answer.

- Include physical activity in any dietary program. Besides toning your body, exercise before a meal can help stimulate your appetite. (See Chapter 9 for more about exercise.)
- Consider the fact that your appetite may vary based on how you feel on any given day. During times when you're feeling better, make sure that you eat all the nutrient-packed foods you can to compensate for those times when you do not feel as well.
- Stay informed! The more you know about the links between diet and health, the better able you'll be to make best use of this enjoyable activity.

A Final Morsel

Before modifying your diet, be sure to speak to your physician or a qualified nutritionist who can offer guidance on what changes are best for you. A good nutritionist understands the biochemistry of the body and can recommend ways to balance it through the use of foods as well as vitamins, minerals, and other dietary supplements. Also keep in mind that although proper diet is an important part of any treatment program—and is almost totally within your control—it is one of the most frequently ignored approaches to health. Good nutrition is *not* an alternative therapy. It is fundamental to everything else you do for your body. While it is sometimes difficult to eat the right foods, isn't it encouraging to know that once you begin to eliminate any harmful foods and increase your intake of nutrient-rich ones, you're sure to feel healthier and more energetic? And you'll benefit from the peace of mind that comes from doing everything you can to help yourself. So eat healthy, eat wisely, and enjoy!

CHAPTER NINE

Rest and Exercise

Two of the most important components of any treatment program for OA are rest and exercise. The proper proportion for you will be determined by your physician or physical therapist, since no two people have the same needs.

Let's discuss these two important factors in more detail.

Rest

Rest is important in the treatment of OA. It is necessary to give your joints and muscles a chance to "recharge their batteries." After resting, you will be better able to maintain an alert, active state.

Regularly scheduled rest periods may help to keep you as strong as possible for the remainder of your day. However, if you often feel very tired, this may be your body's way of telling you that you need additional rest periods. So pay attention to it!

The tricky thing about rest is that, although getting enough is important, too much can be as dangerous as too little. Too much rest may allow your muscles and tendons to become weaker and your joints to get stiffer. If you rest too much, your bones may get even softer. You may feel even more tired. And the more rest you get, the more you want. This creates a vicious cycle.

Rest is vital in learning to live with OA, but it must be properly prescribed. There are differing opinions regarding how long rest periods should be. Some people feel you should schedule several five- to fifteen-minute rest periods per day. Others feel you should schedule two thirty- to sixty-minute rest periods each day. There are plenty of other opinions as well. Your physician will help you to determine which rest periods are most appropriate for you. How? By taking into consideration the severity of your disease, your lifestyle, and other aspects of day-to-day living.

How should you rest? Well, you don't have to lie in bed like a mummy! Just being in a relaxed, comfortable position that places little or no stress on your joints is restful.

Exercise

In the previous section, we saw how extra rest is essential for OA, can help you cope with fatigue, and is important in giving your body a chance to heal and "recharge." But we also saw that too much rest can make you feel more tired, leading to more rest, more fatigue, more rest . . . Well, you get the picture. What's the solution? Exercise! The right types and amounts of exercise can help you break the fatigue-rest-fatigue cycle and make you feel better in countless other ways. In fact, working toward a higher level of fitness is one of the best ways to battle fatigue.

A big problem is that, because of pain, many people with OA are less inclined to exercise. This only accelerates the progression of the disease, because it leads to the loss of cartilage, muscle strength, muscle tone, flexibility, and the range of motion of the joints. Developing a comprehensive exercise program, therefore, is essential.

In this chapter, you'll learn about the many benefits of exercise, and see how you—with the help of your physician or other health-care professional—can design your own personal exercise program.

THE BENEFITS OF EXERCISE

Regular exercise is an essential component of your treatment for OA. What are the benefits of exercise for you? Regular exercise results in better muscle tone and stronger muscles, which in turn improves joint strength and stability. Exercise also improves your posture, coordination, and balance while reducing morning stiffness and the likelihood of developing joint deformities. In some cases, it can even improve the appearance of deformities that already exist. Finally, exercise has a number of well-known benefits that apply to everyone, whether or not they have OA:

- Reduced risk of heart disease and osteoporosis.
- Increased resistance to disease.
- Longer life expectancy.
- Less depression and anxiety.
- Better mental efficiency.
- More relaxation.
- More assertiveness.
- Better attitude about your body.
- Stronger bones—increased bone thickness and mass.
- More restful sleep.
- Higher self-esteem.

Don't you wish that exercise could do all this instantly? Unfortunately, it can't. Exercise must be undertaken regularly, on an ongoing basis, to achieve all these benefits. Make sure, too, that you don't get involved in any exercise that is too strenuous without asking your doctor, nurse, or physical therapist. You want to aid progress, not inhibit it.

Exercise can keep your body trim. And for best health, you should keep your muscles firm, firm, firm, which is better than flabby, flabby, flabby! Exercise benefits your cardiovascular and digestive systems by helping them work more efficiently. As a result, someone who participates in regular exercise usually has more energy, has fewer physical complaints, and sleeps better than someone who is more sedentary. Is that all? Nope! Exercise can also reduce pain and make you feel less fatigued. It has even been named as the closest thing to a "magic bullet" for maintaining youth and optimal health when used in combination with proper nutrition.

Exercise is as good for your psychological well-being as it is for your physical condition. Has your self-esteem been affected as a result of having OA? Exercise can restore some of your confidence in your body and make you feel more capable—more in control. Living with OA may have also increased your level of stress. Exercise is a great release for that stress. For many people, exercise is more calming than a tranquilizer, and it has no untoward side effects. Through exercise, you can let off steam, relieve boredom and frustration, and clear your mind. In fact, virtually any troubling emotion—depression, anger, fear, and anxiety among them—can be controlled, either wholly or partially, through exercise. And if that's not enough of a lure, an exercise program can lead to some healthy social interactions—which are always good for the mind.

SO WHY AREN'T YOU EXERCISING?

Considering all the good things that exercise does, you may wonder why everybody isn't out there getting their motors running. Some people may avoid exercise not because of a lack of desire, but because they find it so tiring. Or they're in so much pain that they fear that exercise will only increase their discomfort. Or perhaps they are afraid that exercise may cause additional problems. While these feelings are understandable, remember that if you become less and less active, your fatigue will only increase and you will have less energy, not more. Why? Because of deconditioning—the weakening of muscles over time due to inactivity.

The good news is that, even if if has already happened, deconditioning can be reversed in time. How? Through exercise! By embarking on a gradually building exercise program, you can slowly increase your ability to participate in more and more activities.

Some people feel that exercise is, at best, extremely boring and, at worst, very unpleasant. Only a small percentage of people really and truly enjoy regular exercise. (Are you one of them?) So the best approach is to focus on exercises—and environments—that are as pleasant as possible.

This will enable you to more easily keep your commitment to your exercise program.

How can you begin? Try to participate in activities that emphasize good muscle tone and do not aggravate your OA. For example, if OA affects your knees or hips, walking or swimming may be better than jogging. It is also important to exercise regularly, rather than exercising only whenever the spirit moves you!

Remember that you need a proper balance between rest and exercise. Too much exercise may do more harm than good because it can cause greater pain and inflammation in your joints. A proper balance of rest and exercise can best be determined by your physician or other health therapist. However, only by trial and error can you really discover whether you are exercising or resting in the proper amounts.

GETTING STARTED

Before beginning any exercise program you should, of course, consult with your physician, who will probably be the one either to prescribe a treatment program or refer you to a physical therapist or exercise trainer. The specifics of your exercise program will depend upon the severity of your OA, the severity of your pain and inflammation, your overall physical condition, the medication you're taking, your day-to-day activities, and the joints that are affected.

Once your physician has approved your program, you must commit yourself to a regular routine. There is no benefit to be gained by exercising for a day or two and then giving up. If you want to feel better, you'll have to exercise regularly. But be patient. Most exercise programs really don't show results for three or four weeks or more. Remember, as long as you stick to your exercise program, you will see results.

Anyone who attempts to accelerate an exercise program to bring about faster results will end up suffering—and, possibly, abandoning it. So implement your exercise program gradually. In fact, the longer it's been since you've done any exercise, the slower your return should be.

Expect the first few weeks of your program to be the most difficult. Why? Because if you haven't been very active lately, you're probably out

of shape. This is not meant as a put-down. Your muscles simply need time
to regain their strength. So expect increased fatigue for a while, as well as
a few new aches and pains. These temporary discomforts are perfectly normal, and will disappear as you consistently participate and gradually increase your exercise. How often must you exercise in order to reap the
many benefits of physical activity? Usually, you must exercise three or
four times a week, for a minimum of twenty minutes each time, in order to
recondition your body. However, some people have found that they feel
best when they exercise five or six times a week. Gradually, you'll find out
what works for you.

EXERCISING CAUTION

I have already mentioned the importance of working with a physician,
physical therapist, or other health-care professional when starting an exercise program. This will not just ensure that the program you've chosen is
safe, but will also give you a partner in your program—someone who will
help you keep track of what you're doing and of how it's helping you. Start
building up your exercise ability gradually. Know your limits and don't do
more than your doctor or therapist has prescribed.

If you're working with a health spa or club, you should, of course, inform the staff of your condition. But remember that they are not health-
care professionals or experts on OA. So be sure to okay any exercise
program recommended by the club with your doctor. If you have had
surgery recently, you may be restricted for a period of time. Find out what
you can do as an alternative so that you regain your strength and don't take
two steps back.

Be careful when you exercise. If you exercise a weak joint, you may
run the risk of further damaging the joint. Therefore, although exercise
doesn't necessarily have to stop if specific joints are weak, it should focus
either on joints that aren't affected or very carefully (and minimally) on
joints that are.

We mentioned earlier that you should expect to feel more aches and
pains as you begin your program. But it's important to learn the difference
between muscle soreness, which is probably a normal response to exer-

cise, and acute pain. Acute pain may mean that you're overdoing it, or that you're participating in an exercise that's a no-no. The old saying "No pain, no gain" is not true when you have a condition such as OA. So if the discomfort you feel is extreme, by all means stop exercising and consult with a professional. You may have to choose a different form of exercise or otherwise modify your routine.

It's probably not a good idea to participate in high-tension exercises, such as weight lifting or ball-squeezing. Nor should you become involved in sports involving jerky motions, such as tennis, bowling, or golf. Not only do these require strength that you may not have, but they may put too much immediate pressure on those joints that you don't want to stress. Jogging is another activity that you may wish to avoid, especially if OA is causing your knees to become sore or swollen.

It is also vital to make sure that when you do exercise, you do it properly, following appropriate guidelines and safety rules. Again, do not build up your pace too quickly. You'll want to follow a concept in exercise known as the *progression principle*. This principle states that exercise should be started slowly and, as time goes by, increased in intensity.

One last caution is in order. Sometimes the pain of OA can be so uncomfortable that you may not be able to do any exercise at all. Don't feel guilty about this, and don't try to force yourself to exercise when you're really not up to it. Rest as long as necessary, and be assured that you will be able to exercise eventually.

TYPES OF EXERCISE

While all exercises can be used to improve stamina and muscle tone, different types have other aims as well. It is these other goals that determine the category into which a particular exercise falls. How many categories are there? Most exercises belong in one of four groups: stretching exercises, range-of-motion exercises, aerobic exercises, and muscle-strengthening exercises. Which type should you choose? Well, it's usually important to include exercises that will maintain and build muscle tone, normal joint motion, and overall fitness. So you will probably want to incorporate a few different types of exercises—stretching and aerobics, for example—into your program. Of course, your choice will depend partly on your own specific needs and partly on your own preferences.

Once you have chosen the exercises for your program, you will want to be sure to perform them in a particular order each time you do your routine. Most routines, for example, begin with a warm-up, which uses stretching exercises to ready you for more vigorous activity; proceed to the main part of the routine—the aerobics, for instance; and end with a cool-down period. This sequence helps prevent injury, and leaves you feeling exhilarated at the end of the routine.

Let's look at the four different categories, and see what each type can do for you. Remember, though, that more important than the type of exercise you do is the regularity with which you perform your exercise routine. Consistency and persistence are the keys to improving your strength, endurance, flexibility, and general well-being. And combining regular exercise with proper nutrition makes good sense.

Stretching Exercises

If you are inactive and do not use your joints properly, you become less flexible and can even experience muscle cramps. In fact, when joints are stiff, even the smallest motion can cause pain. Stretching exercises help to eliminate stiffness or tightness in the muscles, tendons, and ligaments surrounding the joints, relieving pain and preventing injury. Stretching exercises are a great way to begin any exercise routine because they strengthen muscles, improve circulation, and increase flexibility.

Certain "positioning" exercises can be very helpful for someone with OA. Hips, knees, hands, and shoulders are particularly vulnerable to OA. By stretching your body into certain positions, you may be able to help yourself avoid some OA-related deformities. Examples of positioning exercises include reaching for a high spot on a wall or door and stretching out on your bed.

Where can you learn stretching exercises? If you belong to an exercise club, the instructors will certainly be able to show you some gentle, effective ones. Just make sure that they know about your OA and any other problems, and that they are competent to advise you. And, of course, numerous exercise books and videotapes are available for people at all levels of proficiency.

Range-of-Motion Exercises

Range of motion describes the way a joint moves in different directions. OA can reduce the range of motion possible in a particular joint. A range-of-motion exercise helps maintain or increase a joint's complete movement by moving a body part as far as possible in every direction. These exercises, therefore, are especially important in treatment for OA.

Range-of-motion exercises increase the joint's ability to move in various directions by manipulating the muscles attached to them. Examples include raising your arms above your head, or spreading and stretching your fingers apart. Range-of-motion exercises that are involved in OA may be very helpful in preventing loss of mobility, restoring lost movement, reducing stiffness, and, hopefully, preventing deformity in the joints. They are usually done daily.

Extend and move your arms in a wide circular motion. There you have an example of range-of-motion exercise. You do need to be flexible to perform these exercises, so be sure to stretch before you begin. Like all other exercises, range-of-motion routines can be learned through books and videotapes, or from the staff of your local gym.

Aerobic Exercises

By definition, an aerobic exercise (also called an endurance exercise) is one that involves or improves oxygen consumption by requiring increased amounts of oxygen for prolonged periods of time. These type of exercises are less beneficial for specific joints, but more helpful for overall fitness. Doing aerobic exercise for at least twenty minutes per session, a minimum of three times a week, can strengthen your heart, improve circulation, reduce blood pressure, and relieve tension. So aerobic exercises can give you more energy, improve your endurance, and make you feel a whole lot happier, too.

However, when beginning your exercise program, be careful not to overdo. Depending on your treatment and your current level of fitness, consider starting with a sustained five- or ten-minute effort. Then gradually increase this time as you feel stronger and have more confidence.

What are some examples of aerobic activities? Aerobic exercises include brisk walking, step exercises, jogging, riding a regular or stationary bicycle, climbing stairs, using a treadmill, aerobic dancing, and swimming. So you see, you don't have to belong to a gym or buy a videotape to enjoy aerobics! Heel-to-toe walking is a style of walking that involves your whole body in one gliding, heart-pumping, joint-flexing, muscle-working, calorie-burning motion.

Is aerobic exercise for you? Everybody can certainly benefit from the many advantages it has to offer. And aerobic activities are a good complement to stretching, strengthening, and range-of-motion exercises.

Muscle-Strengthening Exercises

Strengthening exercises are important because they build up strength in the muscles and other tissues that support the joints and keep them stable. These exercises also help maintain the strength that you already have, and are especially important if you have experienced any decrease in muscle strength.

There are two types of strengthening (or muscle-tightening) exercises that may be helpful to you. Isometric exercises are strengthening exercises that do not involve any movement within the joints. These involve pushing one immovable force against another. You strongly tighten the muscle but do not move the joint. As a result, strength can be improved without further stressing the joints. Trying to pull your hands apart after firmly clasping them together, or pushing the palm of one hand against the palm of the other, are both isometrics. Isometric exercises are convenient in that they can be done anywhere—in the car, in a chair, even in bed. And although you won't be moving around, you'll still be giving your muscles a great workout.

The other type of strengthening exercises are resistive exercises, which actively move the joint against something that offers resistance, such as a weight, or against other objects. Because there is less chance of straining an already fragile joint, isometric exercises are usually considered safer than resistive exercises.

Where can you learn some appropriate muscle-strengthening exercises? Again, libraries, bookstores, video stores, and your local gym are likely to be your best resources.

ACTIVE VERSUS PASSIVE EXERCISE

You can also categorize different types of exercise as *active* or *passive*. If you are moving your body without anyone else helping you, you're doing active exercise. If you're moving it and someone is helping you, these are assisted active exercises. If you relax while a physical therapist, family member, or friend moves your joints (which may happen when you've had a severe flare-up), then you're doing passive exercise.

GENERAL EXERCISE GUIDELINES

It is good to keep in mind a few general guidelines that will help you derive the greatest benefits from your exercise program—without straining your muscles or worsening your symptoms. Some of the following points have not yet been mentioned in this chapter. Others have already been discussed, but they are important enough that they bear repeating.

- Don't feel that you have to wait until you feel better before starting your exercise program. Starting sooner may help you to feel better more quickly. But get professional advice and supervision.
- Make sure you check with your physician before starting any exercise program. This way, you'll know that the program is right for you. This is especially important if you have had joint replacement surgery or have other medical problems, such as heart disease.
- Begin every exercise routine with a short warm-up. The best warm-ups use stretching exercises to limber the muscles, preparing the body for the more strenuous activities to follow.
- Develop your ability to tolerate exercise slowly. You can improve the way your joints and muscles function by regularly increasing the amount of exercise you do, but do this gradually. Too rapid an increase or too intense an exercise program may only worsen the pain

you are experiencing—and lessen your desire to exercise. It may also damage the very joints that you want to protect and improve.

- If you experience a lot of pain or inflammation in your joints, do your exercises with much more caution. Isometric exercises may be helpful. Very gentle range-of-motion exercises may also be suggested. Avoid exercising tender, inflamed, or injured joints.

- If you feel intense pain, stop exercising. You may have overdone it. If your pain persists for more than a few days, report this to your doctor.

- Anticipate minor discomfort during your first days or weeks of exercising. Remember, you're moving joints that may not want to be moved! Bending a joint and stretching the surrounding muscles, tendons, and ligaments may cause some pain. It's a good idea to push a joint actually a little beyond the level at which pain first occurs. This helps to increase joint mobility. Applying heat before exercising may help to relax tense muscles and reduce pain. But if you experience too much discomfort or pain, or if it lasts for a long time, cut back. It may indicate that you're overdoing it. Always listen to your body!

- Exercise at the time of day when you have the least pain and stiffness. But rather than exercising whenever the spirit moves you, set aside a regular time each day or several days a week for your exercise routine. Then stick to your schedule!

- Initially, commit yourself to your exercise program for at least two months. By that time you will probably be able to see the benefits of the program, and will be motivated to continue. This will decrease the chances of your becoming an exercise dropout.

- Aim to do as much exercise as possible on your own, even though you may initially need the help of either a family member or a physical therapist.

- If you experience muscle cramps, tightness, or discomfort after exercise, treat yourself to a hot bath, a massage, or a sauna, and drink plenty of water.

- Don't compare your exercise program to somebody else's. You wouldn't compare your doses or types of medication to somebody else's, would you? (Nor should you!) Remember that your own situation—your special needs and limits—is unique.

A FINAL EXERCISE

Exercise can be either extremely valuable or extremely harmful—or anything in between—depending on the care you use in choosing and following your program. Because every person is different, there is no one set of exercises that can be recommended for everyone. But everybody is capable of doing some exercise, and everybody can benefit from them. Just don't jump in feet first. Use your head. Speak to your physician—or perhaps to a physical therapist who is in touch with your physician. Then start slowly, build up your stamina, and enjoy your improved health!

CHAPTER TEN

Activities

What can you do, what can't you do? Sure, you have OA, but what does this mean in terms of the basic activities in your life? What *can* you do and what *can't* you do? Even if you feel wonderful, you will still want to curtail any vigorous activities. You don't want to put any strain on your joints.

As I've said many times before, each person is unique. The kinds of things you did before beginning treatment for OA can influence what you can or want to do now. Your current physical condition is also a determining factor. For example, if you've had joint replacement surgery, you'll want to hold off on most exertions until healing has taken place and your doctor has given you the green light (or even a cautious yellow) to continue. So let's discuss some of the more important types of activities that people participate in.

Activities of Daily Living

Among the things you do each day are numerous routine tasks—the activities of daily living (ADL). But there's a problem. The pain and reduced mobility of OA may limit these activities. This can be frustrating. Prior to being diagnosed, you may have taken such simple tasks for granted. The difficulties you may be experiencing now, however, may make you irritated, even depressed and upset, rather than enthusiastic about trying to conquer the problem.

What if you can't do what you want to do? You may not want to ask for help. You may feel that it takes away some of your dignity. This can make you very uncomfortable. However, the future can be brighter. In a very short period of time, you can reorganize your lifestyle, your household, your work environment, and your ADLs in a way that can enable you to do more of what you'd like to do, and feel better about yourself at the same time.

So what ADL difficulties might you have? You may have problems getting dressed or undressed. You may have difficulty with bathroom activities, such as bathing and using the toilet. You may have difficulty applying enough pressure on a washcloth to adequately clean a part of your body. You may have problems holding a toothbrush or comb, or washing and drying various parts of your body. You may have difficulty turning handles and opening doors. You may have trouble opening jars or holding objects that require fine motor coordination. You may have difficulty preparing or eating food. You may have difficulty moving, walking, or going up or down the stairs. Not all people with OA experience these problems. But if you do, you should know that you're not alone, and that there are things you can do to improve the situation?

Modifying your lifestyle or your home is not the same as giving in to OA. Rather, these changes will help you learn how to live most effectively and cope most successfully with your condition.

SIMPLIFY YOUR TASKS

When learning to cope with ADLs, keep in mind that your goal is to make daily living as easy as possible in order to conserve energy and increase your comfort. There are three main reasons for trying to make daily living as easy as possible. You want to protect your joints, relieve pain, and conserve your energy. You will want to reduce or eliminate those activities that aren't necessary, and simplify those that are. This will leave you with more energy for the things you need—or want—to do.

In many cases, various health-care professionals will be able to help you solve any problems you may experience when performing ordinary tasks. But it can also be very satisfying to develop your own solutions to these problems. Of course, any questions you have can be bounced off physicians, physical therapists, or occupational therapists. In fact, one of the occupational therapist's main goals is to help you solve any problems in daily living, especially those at home or related to your occupation. This will greatly improve your overall functioning.

How can you start? Well, begin by evaluating everything you do on a day-to-day basis. Then see how you can make every single thing you do easier. Is this taking the lazy way out? Of course not. You're simply recognizing that every bit of energy you save in the performance of one activity will give you more energy with which to do something else. In addition, conserving your energy is an important way to help you to reduce stress in your joints. It can also help you to reduce much of the fatigue you may experience because of OA.

There are lots of things you can do to help yourself with daily living. Here are some specific suggestions:

- Reorganize your home to make movement easier, and put things within easy reach. For example, you can replace small handles on drawers with bigger ones. You can lubricate drawers so that they open and close more easily. There are a number of different types of gadgets that will make life easier for you.
- Wear clothing that is easier to get on and off.
- Learn how to moderate your activities. Plan them out carefully and pace yourself. Figure out exactly how and when you're going to do each task, what supplies or equipment you're going to need, and how much time you can spend doing them in between rest periods. Planning will help you to reduce the amount of strain, both physical and emotional, that you may experience, and will keep you from getting overtired. You may want to chart all of your activities (required ones, as well as social and leisure activities), to help you to become better organized so that you can pace yourself more effectively.

- Try to reduce the amount of energy you expend in performing any activity. Eliminate any unnecessary activity.

- Improve your time-management skills. Your local library and bookstores should have some excellent books on time management. Many of the tips in these books make such good sense that you'll probably wonder why you didn't think of them yourself! And every bit of time you save will be a big plus.

- Modify any pain-inducing activities as much as possible. If you've already reduced a task to the bare minimum and absolutely can't do anything more about it, put a limit on how much pain you're going to let yourself endure. In general, you may want to avoid pain that lasts longer than fifteen to twenty minutes (but speak to your doctor about this to make sure).

- Use any assistance devices or equipment that you can to conserve energy and protect your joints. Rest intermittently, frequently, and whenever needed. You'll then be able to do more of what you want or need to do. And you'll accomplish it in a healthier way.

USE SUPPORT DEVICES WHEN NECESSARY

There are many different types of support and self-help devices that can help you in your daily activities. Support devices can be resting devices (which are used when you're not doing anything and are designed to immobilize affected joints), functional devices (which are used when you're doing something to strengthen or protect joints that need protections), and corrective devices (which are used when you are inactive, but are designed to strengthen, relieve, or correct a problem).

Any support devices that you purchase or develop should meet certain requirements. They should be durable, lightweight, economical, pleasing to the eye, versatile, and most important, useful.

The support devices that you may find most helpful in daily living fall into five main categories: (1) bath and toilet aids (such as raised toilet seats, handles, bath or shower seats, and rubber mats); (2) dressing aids (such as clothing with Velcro fasteners instead of buttons, shoes that are easier to get on, hooks and pull strings for pulling up zippers, etc.); (3) walking aids (such as canes, crutches, walking sticks, and other support devices; (4) eating aids (such as special long-handled or thick-handled utensils; and (5) household aids (such as book rests, groping tools, and jar openers).

There are many helpful tools and devices available in each category. Detailed information about all of the different types of devices available is beyond the scope of this book. To find out more about specific devices you can use, you may want to consult the Arthritis Foundation or other sources of support. The Arthritis Foundation publishes a self-help manual that includes types of devices, costs, and additional resources designed to help solve many of the different problems with daily living. (See Resource Groups section of this book.)

You can buy many beneficial support devices from surgical supply companies, pharmacies, and health service organizations (who may also have booklets describing the devices), or even borrow many of them from hospitals or volunteer agencies. Remember that any special devices needed to make your home "OA-suitable" may be tax-deductible because of your condition. Obtain a prescription from your physician for any necessary equipment in case it's necessary when filing your income tax returns.

So how do you deal with the fact that you may not be thrilled about using these support devices? Using a cane, crutch, splint, or any other device is *not* a defeat or giving in to OA. It is *not* a sign of weakness. These devices do not lead to dependency; rather, they allow *in*dependence! Don't be embarrassed to use a cane, splint, or brace if doing so speeds up activities, permits you to participate in activities that may have previously been too difficult for you, and helps you to rest and protect your joints. Tell yourself how much your assistive devices are helping you. After all, using one of these devices to help your joints is the same kind of thing as using eyeglasses to help you see properly!

Work

Working can be very important for you. Besides being a source of income (you can't overlook that!), working will make you feel as if your life is proceeding as usual. You may be concerned (an understatement!) if your OA threatens the possibility of working. This may interfere with your financial security.

Even though you have OA, you'll probably want to do as much of what you used to do as possible. Are you afraid that you'll feel like less of a person if you have to stop working? Beyond supplying income, work is important because it helps you to feel independent and gives you a sense of fulfillment. And it often provides a social life and human contact.

Many people question whether they should work if they have OA. If you want to, and you need to, and you can, then you should! You may have to make some modifications, because you don't want to chance putting too much stress on your joints. This would only increase your pain and discomfort, and could cause further damage.

Focusing on five basic issues may help you when you are thinking about working:

1. Do you feel comfortable doing the job? Do you feel physically and emotionally capable? Is it something you want to do? Your condition may have made you more aware of your mortality. As a result, you might decide to start doing something you really want to do!
2. Does your employer still want you to work there? Or will a new employer hire you, given your present physical condition? Should you even say anything about it? (More about this in a later chapter.)
3. Will your colleagues accept you? (Of course, they will not necessarily even notice your condition.)
4. Will your condition affect your attendance at work or your punctuality? If so, will this cause any difficulties on the job?
5. How much stress is involved? Stress is something you definitely want to minimize. You may decide to change jobs if you recognize that your current job is too stressful.

WHAT IF PAIN OR OTHER DISCOMFORTS ARE A PROBLEM?

You may be concerned that symptoms or treatment side effects will prevent you from adequately performing on the job. Certainly, OA can cause pain and other problems, and this may affect your productivity—especially if your treatment is not controlling your pain as well as you'd like it to. OA may cause you to experience fatigue, depression, and adjustment problems. This may affect your work productivity, especially if your treatment has not been as helpful as you may like. Your work rate may slow down, you may be absent more often, and your value to your employer may decrease. You simply may not feel physically able to work. You may get tired easily, and feel that you just don't have the stamina necessary to complete your job satisfactorily. You may need to be off your feet more, or you may have been told not to walk up and down stairs. If your employer is aware of any of these problems, you may be afraid that your value will be questioned—that your job will be in jeopardy.

What can you do? Build up your stamina slowly. Pacing yourself is probably the most important thing you can do. Take frequent rest breaks whenever necessary—and possible—to recharge your batteries. Don't expect too much all at once. If you're not sure how much you can do, do what you can and let the amount of pain in your body be your guide.

There's no reason to believe that once medication and other components of your treatment program begin to help, you won't be able to continue working. On the other hand, even if you can't succeed at your old job because of its requirements, you still may be able to succeed at another job that requires less physical exertion.

SHOULD YOU DISCUSS YOUR CONDITION WITH YOUR EMPLOYER?

What's the best approach if you find you may have to shorten your hours or modify your work in some way? Well, be aware that under the provisions of the Americans with Disabilities Act, employers are now required by law to make "reasonable accommodations" for employees with disabilities. You still have to do what your job description requires, and the precise meaning of the phrase "reasonable accommodations" may be subject to some debate. But if you are a valued employee, your employer will probably be willing to make any feasible modifications necessary to retain your services.

Of course, you may feel uncomfortable about approaching your employer to find out if any changes can be made. It may bother you to seek "special treatment." But consider that any necessary modifications may be small in comparison to the ones your employer would face if he or she had to hire someone to replace you!

What if your employer refuses or is unable to bend the rules? What if you are given an ultimatum that if your productivity does not improve, you will be discharged? If this happens, simply do the best you can. If your employer is not sensitive to your need to pace yourself, and shows little or no willingness to cooperate, then you're probably better off not working there.

You should be aware that, in some cases, even if your employer is willing to accommodate you, union rules and state labor regulations can restrict an employer from making exceptions. In some states, hourly employees cannot make up lost hours except within a certain time frame or those hours are considered overtime. There may also be restrictions on comp time for salaried employees.

What if another employee resents any special treatment you've been given? Try to sit down, one on one, and have a conversation with your unhappy colleague. Explain your situation as much as necessary. Often, this is all that's needed to bring about greater understanding and cooperation. If your coworker still doesn't understand, content yourself with knowing that you tried. Now it's his problem! (More information on dealing with colleagues appears in Chapter 22.)

WHAT IF YOU HAVE TO CHANGE JOBS?

If you are experiencing limitations, your old position may no longer be right for you. If this is the case, you should certainly consider transferring to another job, even if it means getting additional training.

Larry, age 59, had been working in construction all his life. But doctors felt he shouldn't continue this type of work because it was too strenuous for him. It put too much pressure on his joints. Larry became very depressed. He didn't know what else he could do. He shut down emotionally in order to avoid facing the prospect of not being able to work. He feared that his age would be an obstacle. He was even afraid that he didn't have the ability to go out and get new training.

Certainly the prospect of having to look for work is more daunting to some people than it is to others. But if for any reason you are unable to continue in your present job, don't despair. There are many ways you can get the training you need to move into a different position. Your first step might be to check with any of the government services that offer vocational counseling. Counselors in these offices will work with you to determine your aptitude for different jobs. You will then be able to get the training and support you need to find employment in another field. Your State Employment Services may be a good place to start. These services are available free of charge, and may guide you in locating jobs that will match your abilities and limitations. In addition, the Federal Rehabilitation Act of 1973 requires states to include individuals in vocational rehabilitation programs if their previous jobs are no longer appropriate for them. These programs vary, so it's important to check with your state's Office of Vocational Rehabilitation to find out what's available. Any financial adviser you're working with should also be able to help you in this regard.

You may feel that, for financial reasons, you should postpone looking for a new job until your old one has been terminated. This tactic has its pros and cons. If you receive unemployment benefits for losing your job, this could ease your financial burden. But if subsequent employers are reluctant to hire you because of the grounds for your dismissal, this tactic may explode in your face. You are the only one who can decide which course of action is best for your unique needs.

IS WORKING YOUR ONLY OPTION?

As you know, there are many benefits to working, including satisfaction, pride, and money. But a paying job is not the only type of gratifying work that's available. Many meaningful, productive activities can be pursued on a voluntary basis. Check with nonprofit charities, religious and political groups, hospitals, schools, senior-citizen centers, and the like. These organizations, and many more, can always use some extra help. For example, working with a group like the Arthritis Foundation makes many people feel that they are fighting arthritis through helping others with the disease. Volunteer work may even allow you to explore new areas of interest you previously couldn't pursue due to work commitments. And this will help you feel good about yourself in the bargain.

What if you just don't want to work? If this is your preference, and you're able to manage without a job, that's great. But don't use your condition as an excuse for not working. Instead, try to find out what's really bothering you, and explore ways to cope with these issues.

Recreation

By all means, continue to pursue the activities you've always enjoyed, as much as you're physically able. Why? Depending on their nature, recreational activities may help keep you limber and vigorous and even offer pain relief. Just as important, they will provide a welcome diversion from any worries, prevent boredom and depression, and, very likely, put you in contact with other people.

Many people with OA participate in a wide variety activities, including boating, swimming, skating, golf, tennis, dancing—the list goes on and on. What you do or don't do depends solely on your own condition and, of course, on the recommendations of your doctor. If you try an activity without experiencing pain, swelling, or lasting discomfort, you're probably okay. On the other hand, there may be times when you feel that your condition keeps you from doing certain things. However, if your doctor approves of an activity, at least you know that you can try it. It's up to you and your doctor to decide which activities are best for you.

You're probably participating in exercises to increase muscle strength and maintain the range of motion in your joints. The exercises that are found in normal hobbies and other types of pleasurable activities can actually be extensions of these exercises. This is what falls under the category of therapeutic recreation, and the advantage is that not only are these exercises important for joint mobility, but they're also fun!

Why is it so helpful to participate in activities that you enjoy? One reason is that they can improve your ability to take care of yourself. They can help promote and maintain your participation in the normal activities of daily living. They can certainly enhance your social life and improve your spirits as well. And because they're enjoyable, you're more likely to spend time doing them.

Travel

If you think you might like to travel, discuss it with your physician first. Chances are that if you're able to get around your own neighborhood without assistance, you can probably handle traveling with confidence. If you do have difficulty getting around, you'll want to be more selective about where you go. Some people opt to use wheelchairs to protect their joints, as well as to increase the distance they can travel. Using a wheelchair might not be a bad idea for these people. But others are afraid of being seen in a wheelchair, or are even more afraid that once they use them, they'll be "stuck" in them forever. Neither of these fears is valid, but both can interfere with happy travel plans. The truth shall set you free—free to travel!

Do all individuals with OA avoid traveling? No. Some don't travel simply because they feel it's too expensive. This may have nothing to do with OA. But plenty of others do travel, whether their trips are short or long. Some travel simply to prove to themselves that they can. As with any other aspect of living with your OA, planning ahead and taking the proper precautions can allow you to travel with a free mind (although not with free airfare!) How should you plan ahead for a vacation? Let's explore some of the things you should do.

When making hotel reservations or arranging other accommodations, make sure that they fit your needs. For example, you'll want to know where you can get proper medical care, if necessary. Compile a list of clinics, hospitals, and physicians in the parts of the world where you may be traveling. In addition, find out if there is a local chapter of the Arthritis Foundation at your destination.

TAKE MEDICATIONS AND OTHER SUPPLIES

One of your biggest concerns about traveling may be: What happens if I run out of sufficient medication or other supplies? There are two things you can do. First, have extra medication, equipment, and supplies packed in case any unexpected situations arise. Second, ask your physician to write up extra prescriptions to take with you. At least you'll be prepared if you need more. You may also want to ask if you can keep your doctor "on call," so that you can contact him in case there's an emergency. If you're going to a foreign country, you may want to have the prescription translated into the language of that country in case the pharmacist has difficulty understanding English. What if foreign languages were never your forte? Try checking with a teacher of that particular foreign language in a local school. Check with the airline that travels to that country. Representatives who speak the language will probably be willing to translate for you. As a last resort, you may want to check with the foreign embassy of that particular country. This may take a little extra time, but your mind will be more at ease when you do travel.

If you are flying, carry medication and other necessary supplies with you. Do not pack all supplies in your luggage. If your luggage ends up in Des Moines when you're flying to Miami, you don't want to be left without what you need. Besides, if for any reason you need a pill during the flight, it would be rather inconsiderate of you to ask the flight attendant to climb down into the baggage hold to get it. Leave medication in the original bottles with the labels clearly visible. This will help you get through customs without embarrassing inquiries.

IDENTIFY YOURSELF

It's always a good idea to travel with complete identification, not just for your luggage but for yourself. The Medic Alert bracelet is accepted worldwide as identification of a person with a medical problem. In addition, make sure your wallet contains an identification card with complete details about your condition, the type of medication you need, and any other pertinent information. Again, if you're going to a foreign country, make sure that this information is translated into the language of that country.

AIR TRAVEL

Let's say your vacation is set, you're flying to Paradise, and you're now making the final preparations before leaving for the airport. Any special considerations? You bet!

If you have any physical restrictions, discuss these in advance, either with an airline representative or with your travel agent. Airlines frequently have special services for individuals with restricted mobility. For example, you may be able to board early, select your seat in advance, have wheelchair access to and from the gate, and have special meals, if necessary. You may choose to request a bulkhead seat (one found directly behind a cabin divider), which may give you more room to stretch your legs. If you have your own wheelchair and you plan on traveling with it, check with an airline representative to find out what regulations apply.

TRAIN TRAVEL

There is quite a variety of passenger train service throughout the country and abroad. Some trains are very accessible for individuals with disabilities. Others are not as accommodating. If you're thinking of traveling by train, speak with a railroad representative or your travel agent before making a final decision.

CRUISES

More and more cruise ships have special accommodations for people with physical restrictions. Some have rooms specifically designed for individuals with limited mobility. Ramps and wide doorways may be available, too. If you're planning on taking a cruise, make sure that you know what ports of call the ship will be stopping at. In certain Caribbean and Mexican ports, for example, the ship does not dock at the pier. Rather, it drops anchor away from the pier and small boats are used to get you ashore. This may be more difficult for you if you have any physical restrictions. Again, if you're taking your own wheelchair, be sure to find out what regulations may apply.

BUS TRAVEL

Bus travel is becoming easier for people with disabilities. Even if you use a wheelchair, it can probably be stowed and someone can help you get on and off the bus. And newer buses have equipment to board you with your wheelchair.

A FINAL CONFIRMATION

Remember, many individuals with OA feel absolutely no reluctance to travel anywhere. If you haven't traveled recently, you may want to build up your confidence by taking short trips first. Taking a three-month trip around the world might be a bit much. Even an overnight trip might be traumatic. Start with a couple of day trips, then weekend trips, working your way up to short-distance, week-long excursions. Expanding your travel activities slowly is a good way to develop your confidence. There are special travel agencies for people with disabilities. Look in your local Yellow Pages.

Climate Concerns

One major lifestyle change some people with OA consider is moving to a different climate. For years, people have believed that moving to a warm, dry climate could be helpful for OA. It is true that people who retire to such climates, or spend months at a health spa there, may feel better. However, neither the spa nor the climate will necessarily have a significant effect on the course of the disease, although either may be helpful in relieving symptoms. There is no evidence that any specific kind of climate improves or cures osteoarthritis.

Sure, some people like the idea of moving. It may give them a psychological lift. In some cases, people may feel better after moving to other climates. But then again, this is true for people who don't have OA as well.

In order to decide if such a change would benefit you, consider the potential emotional and financial effects. For instance, you'd have to find a place to live, might have to look for a new job, and possibly even need to adopt an entirely new lifestyle. You'll be leaving the familiar, including friends and, possibly, family behind (of course, this may be a blessing in disguise if you're leaving behind people who deserve to be left behind!). Do you have family members, friends, or acquaintances in the proposed new location? If not, are you someone who makes friends easily, or is that something difficult for you? It's important to consider what kind of social outlets and support network you are likely to have after you move. You should also investigate what kinds of important services and resources, from medical facilities to public libraries to shopping areas and more, would be available to you if you were to relocate.

Finally, you have to weigh the advantages of moving (such as the possibility of feeling more comfortable) and the disadvantages (such as disrupting your family). If you really are contemplating a geographical change, it's probably a good idea to take an extended vacation in that location before actually committing yourself to such a move. If a move is going to help you to feel better, you'll probably realize this during your extended vacation. But remember, on a vacation, you usually don't have to cook, clean, or participate in many of the other chores of everyday life. You may feel better only because of less stress and less wear and tear. However, once you move, you'll once again have all the responsibilities you have now, so stress may recur.

And So . . .

By now, you've learned a lot about coping with OA, and you know that staying active is just as important as any other strategy. You want to feel productive and enjoy life. You don't want to let OA confine you to your closet. So don't let it. Certainly you should modify any activities that are causing you discomfort, and you should do only what you physically can do, but the key word is *do*!

CHAPTER ELEVEN

Finances

Having OA can be a pain in the pocketbook! Why? Any chronic illness can be expensive, and OA is no exception. The bills for doctor's visits, laboratory tests, hospitalizations, surgery, medications, and other medical services all add up. Lost earnings, too, may add to the financial burden, for instance, if you find that you can work only part-time, or that you must give up work altogether. The costs of having arthritis total up to billions of dollars each year in the United States. Certainly, the cost for each person—as well as the sources of these costs—varies considerably. But it may not take long for financial security to turn into financial troubles.

What if you can't work, or are only able to hold down a part-time job? Your condition may affect your ability to work. This may cause problems with your job. So it's possible that your employability will be reduced because of your OA. Financial problems may arise from lost earnings or income.

Osteoarthritis can also be costly because of changes at home. You may need to have other people help you, or you may need to make renovations in your home. You may need someone to help around the house, such as a cleaning person. All of these things cost money, adding to your financial burden. As your medical costs rise, your budget becomes tighter and tighter. If costs continue to skyrocket, you may feel like you're being strangled.

Can anything help? Although OA can be an expensive disease, it need not be alarmingly so if you're careful. If you take proper care of yourself and begin treatment as early as possible, you can prevent more serious (and expensive) problems from arising. What else can you do? Let's take a look at the many ways in which you can prevent or ease financial problems as you cope with OA.

Talk to Others

If mounting medical expenses threaten to engulf you, perhaps the first thing you should do is speak to other people with OA. Through a support group, for instance, you may meet others in similar situations. Find out what they have done to control and meet the costs of their own care. Even though you may initially be embarrassed to bring up this subject, the common bond that exists among people with medically induced financial problems should quickly put you at ease. You'll be glad you brought it up!

For more ideas, you might contact your physician, hospital administrators, and other health professionals; social workers; and various organizations, such as the Arthritis Foundation. Through these contacts, you will be able to find out about certain benefits, and how to apply for them. You may be eligible for disability payments (if you have a policy that covers this). Even if you are not poverty-stricken, your medical bills alone may qualify you for medical assistance in the form of Medicaid. You will need to determine the requirements for the state where you live because Medicaid coverage varies.

Lower Your Medication Costs

If your treatment includes medication, the use of generic drugs may save you money. Generic medication is sold by its chemical name rather than the more common brand name, and is usually less expensive. Ask your physician if you can take the generic versions of any drugs you're currently using. If so, your doctor will let your pharmacist know that he has okayed the substitution. Remember, though, that not all generics may have the same therapeutic response as their brand name counterparts.

Some pharmaceutical manufacturers have programs to help make some drugs available free of charge to needy patients. These are known as "indigent patient drug programs" and are available through your physician. To qualify, you must have low income and no health insurance. Your doctor or nurse will contact the pharmaceutical company and request an application which you must complete and then have your doctor authorize. Some states also have programs to assist low-income people with the cost of prescription medications.

Attend a Clinic

If medical costs are overwhelming you, consider attending a clinic rather than a private physician for medical care. Because clinics usually operate on a sliding-fee schedule, you may be able to receive medical care at a reduced cost. In some cases, you may even be able to continue seeing the physician who's treating you now, since many physicians see patients in hospital clinics as well as in their offices. A physician may not accept your insurance in his office but you could be treated by that same doctor in an alternative setting, such as a hospital outpatient center.

How can you locate a good clinic in your area? Your local hospital or your physician should be able to guide you to one that has the resources you need.

Insurance Can Be an Assurance

Health insurance coverage is essential. Many people have at least some of their medical costs defrayed by insurance. However, certain costs may not be covered by some insurance policies. That's all the more reason to get the best insurance coverage possible. But what happens if you run out of money or insurance, or if your coverage is not good enough? Most insurance policies have a deductible—an amount of money that you must pay before the insurance coverage begins. In addition, you may have to pay a small percentage of all costs (known as coinsurance or a copayment), with the insurance company picking up the rest of the tab.

Because you have a chronic illness, you may have more difficulty getting either life or health insurance. Speak to a reputable insurance agent and find out exactly what you are entitled to. Also speak with a social worker to learn what your community offers in the way of aid.

GETTING THE MOST FROM YOUR INSURANCE POLICY

If you have a health insurance policy, contact your agent or company benefits manager as soon as possible and find out as much as you can about the benefits. (The policy itself will provide this information, too, of course.) It is important to know the amount of your deductible; the number of covered hospital days and the amount paid per day; how much coverage you have for surgery and anesthesia; how much coverage you have for physical therapy—both inpatient and outpatient—should that be necessary; whether the company will pay for second opinions; and what your maximum lifetime coverage is. Also, make sure you know all of the procedures necessary to obtain a referral, file a claim, and submit an appeal.

How can you help ensure that the process of claim filing and reimbursement runs smoothly? If you are responsible for paying your own insurance premiums, make sure you pay them on time. Don't allow your policy to lapse. Also, be sure to keep track of paperwork. Every time you send in a claim, keep copies of the claim form and of any doctors' bills for your own files. These may prove invaluable if a problem arises in the processing of your claim. If, in fact, you do not receive reimbursement within sixty days, follow up by phone or letter, and request an explanation if the company has denied payment. If you don't receive a satisfactory response, contact the insurance commissioner of your state, requesting an investigation.

Also, keep records of the amount your insurance company pays on each claim, as well as what you pay. Your out-of-pocket payments may be deductible on your next income-tax return. (Your accountant should be able to provide more information on this.)

WHAT IF YOU LEAVE YOUR JOB?

In the past, when people left jobs (voluntarily or otherwise), they also lost the health insurance that was included with that job. In that regard, a federal law called the Consolidated Omnibus Budget Reconciliation Act (COBRA) now can be very helpful. Under this plan, your employer has to allow you to keep your existing health insurance policy, with the same coverage, for up to eighteen months after you leave. You will have to pay for this coverage, and it is likely to cost you more than it did when you were working, but it's better than not having any insurance. Many people are concerned about the stance of insurance companies regarding preexisting conditions. But as long as you have already been covered for OA, you will be able to get coverage from subsequent insurance companies, as long as you don't let your coverage lapse.

WHAT IF YOUR INSURANCE IS INADEQUATE?

What happens if your health coverage is exhausted, or if your insurance is simply not good enough? Well, you may be able to increase the ceiling for your coverage. Additional insurance may also be available for so-called catastrophic medical expenses. Be aware, though, that people with chronic illnesses may have difficulty obtaining additional health or disability insurance. However, a good insurance agent can work with you to get any exclusions time-reduced with supporting medical documentation. Don't give up! It's important to fight any insurance discrimination, whether it takes the form of canceled coverage, reduced benefits, increased premiums, or loss of insurance due to employment termination.

WHAT IF YOU HAVE NO HEALTH INSURANCE?

If you are not currently covered by health insurance, you will want to immediately contact all your resources—your accountant, your lawyer, your financial adviser, and organizations such as the Arthritis Foundation, for instance—to learn about available options. The more individuals you contact, the more likely it is that you'll find the information you need. Of course, if you are unable to obtain coverage and can't afford to pay your medical costs, you may be able to obtain assistance from government programs.

Government Programs May Help

Some government insurance programs may be very important sources of financial support. You may be covered (at least to some degree) by Medicare, where eligibility is determined by age, chronic disability, or both; Medicaid, where benefits vary from state to state; or social security disability insurance. Let's discuss these different government programs, what they do, and how you can participate (if you're eligible).

MEDICARE

Medicare, a federal health insurance program, provides coverage for Americans age sixty-five and over, and for disabled people of any age who qualify for and receive social security disability insurance (SSI). The degree of coverage provided by Medicare varies widely, so it's vital for you to determine exactly what health services Medicare will cover in your case.

There are two components to the Medicare Program. Part A covers hospitalization costs as well as inpatient services in a skilled nursing facility, home health services, and hospice care. The second part, Part B, covers doctors' charges, outpatient hospital services (including physical therapy), and specified medical items and services not covered under Part A. Unlike Part A, it is voluntary, and requires you to enroll and pay a monthly premium. In addition, Part B requires an annual deductible and a 20-percent copayment on your part.

Enrollment in Medicare is automatic upon your application for monthly social security benefits at age sixty-five. If you decide to continue working past the age of sixty-five, you must apply separately for Medicare.

Remember, though, that while Medicare does provide coverage for large costs, it will not cover everything. Especially in the case of a major illness, supplementary medical coverage is vital.

MEDICAID

Medicaid can offer benefits to individuals who are unable to pay for health care. This public assistance program is administered on the state or local level. Who qualifies for Medicaid? Individuals who demonstrate need (that is, people with very low incomes and high medical expenses) may be eligible. If you have any questions about qualifications, or about the benefits themselves, check with your state office of health services for further information.

SOCIAL SECURITY (DISABILITY)

If you are unable to work because of your OA, you may be eligible for disability benefits, which are included in the Social Security Act. The Social Security Disability Program is a federal government program. It is administered and run by the Social Security Administration.

You may experience all kinds of legal problems trying to get these benefits because of the many different definitions of disability. An individual is considered to be disabled if unable to do any substantial gainful work due to a physical or mental impairment; and if the physical or mental condition is expected to last, or has lasted, for at least twelve months or is expected to result in death.

If you are eligible for these benefits, you will receive a fixed monthly benefit, calculated the same way—and equaling the same amount—as your retirement benefits. Your local social security office should be able to tell you if you're eligible for disability insurance. The Arthritis Foundation can also provide important tips if you are thinking of applying for disability.

$umming Up

Financial concerns can be a big worry for people with OA. But there are always things you can do. The earlier you start planning, and the more qualified professionals you consult, the greater the likelihood that medical costs will not become a major problem for you. Hopefully, the variety of insurance coverages available to you will increase, more provisions will be made for meeting your expenses, and requirements and application procedures will become more humane. You want to fight for your rights—and for your dollars. You will then be able to concentrate on your most important goal: living successfully with OA.

PART THREE

Your Emotions

CHAPTER TWELVE

Coping with Your Emotions: An Introduction

How happy are you about having OA? Well, each person's emotional responses to OA are different. Even your own reactions to OA will vary from time to time. The more severe your reactions are, the more they will interfere with your ability to cope.

When first diagnosed, some people scarcely react at all. Either it may not seem real to them or the diagnosis may not even bother them because they've been living with discomfort or pain for so long. But others go through a hard time. Emotional reactions to OA are not always rational. As a matter of fact, in many cases they may be completely irrational!

Your emotions can be like a roller coaster. You may feel okay sometimes and very upset at other times. Emotional ups and downs are very common. But one of the most important aspects of being able to cope with OA is the ability to control your emotions.

Your emotional reactions to OA may start even before treatment begins. Of course, your reaction will depend partly on how suddenly you found out about your health problem. For example, if, with very few warning symptoms, having only recently experienced some pain, you were suddenly diagnosed with OA, you might have a harder time adjusting than if you had been in pain for a while and suspected that a problem existed. Other factors also help shape your response.

Factors Shaping Your Emotional Reactions

A number of factors may play a role in determining how you react to OA. Keep in mind, though, that because there are so many factors, no one can predict just how a person will react at any given time.

How did you generally handle problems before your osteoarthritis was diagnosed? What was your general coping style? Were you calm or nervous? Were you persistent or did you give up easily? Were you successful in coping with stress? How did you handle pain? The way you've handled life's problems in general will suggest how well you will cope with OA and its treatment, and help you identify which areas you'll want to improve.

Your age also has a bearing on how you respond emotionally. What kind of lifestyle have you enjoyed? What was your general physical health prior to the onset of OA? These factors also have a bearing on how you respond emotionally. And what about your relationships? In many cases, your emotional reactions may reflect the responses of significant people in your life. For example, if family members or friends are anxious about your medical condition, this may have an impact on the way you feel.

Which Emotional Reactions?

Do you like yourself less with osteoarthritis? Has your self-image suffered? Any loss of self-esteem can have a very unpleasant effect. You may not feel or behave like yourself. You'll want to deal with this right away in order to return to effective, efficient functioning.

Have you been experiencing anger because you have to go through all this? Are you angry that your joints may never be the same, and that your life may change because of this? Are you worried that you'll always be in pain? Are you afraid of the medication you may need? Do you become depressed when you compare your present life with the way things were? Are you afraid of not being able to cope? Many people living with OA experience feeling depressed, frightened, guilty, and angry. Feeling this way doesn't mean that you are weak. Rather, it means that you are normal! Because of the importance of coping with these and other emotions, a separate chapter has been devoted to each. But other than these specific emotional responses, what else might you be experiencing?

You may become somewhat disoriented. One of the most frightening feelings is that you're not yourself. Experiencing pain can be frightening as well. You may wonder what is happening to your body. It can be reassuring to understand that this happens to many people with OA from time to time. And it can go away.

Managing Emotional Reactions

Because your emotions play such an important role in your life with OA, you'll certainly want to do the best possible job you can of handling them. How? Let's discuss some of the more important things you can do to help manage your emotions.

GATHER INFORMATION

Always stay up to date on the latest information on OA and treatment options, and on any other facts that may be helpful to you. Learn as much as you can. Here's a key point: People are usually more afraid of what they don't know than they are of what they do know. You want to become as educated as possible. That will make you best able to help yourself, both in dealing with others and in controlling your own emotional state. Become an expert on all possible treatment options—both the traditional medical and surgical techniques and the alternative therapies. Use your knowledge to find the best-informed health-care professionals whom you trust, and share updated information with them whenever you think it is appropriate.

So how do you do this? Make sure you obtain current, accurate information. The Arthritis Foundation is an excellent resource, because their information is always up to date. Attend support groups and informational meetings because, in all likelihood, other attendees will have varying degrees of access to current, helpful information. If you surf the Web, make sure that the information you review is reputable, either written by knowledgeable professionals or posted by legitimate organizations.

GET THE BEST MEDICAL CARE POSSIBLE

Make sure you're getting the best possible medical care. If you haven't already done so, you'll want to establish a good working relationship with a physician. This involves seeing a doctor who not only has expertise in treating OA and has kept informed of the most up-to-date research, but is also understanding, available, and sympathetic to your emotional needs. You can contact the Arthritis Association, or browse the Internet for sites on OA and centers that specialize in its treatment. (Advice on creating a good relationship with your physician will be covered in Chapter 23.)

LEARN ABOUT MEDICATIONS THAT CAN HELP YOU COPE

A time may come when you find your emotions have become uncomfortably intense. If this happens, you may want to consider medications that can help you cope. A number of medications can be effective in dealing with depression, anxiety, anger, and many other emotional reactions to OA or its symptoms. Antianxiety medication and antidepressants in particular can be helpful. (More about this in Chapter 6.) If you feel that you might benefit from treatments of this type, be sure to discuss the possibility with your doctor.

JOIN A SUPPORT GROUP

Self-help or support groups can be incredibly helpful, and are one of the best sources of support for people with OA. Groups provide a forum for the exchange of feelings and ideas. Perhaps most important, these groups will

show you that you're not alone. And it is much easier to live with a difficult problem when you know that you're not alone. It's helpful to meet new
people, other than family and friends, who know what you're going through
because they've gone through it themselves.

Members of support groups all have a common goal: to learn how to
live as best they can, and to do as much as they possibly can. You'll see
how others handle problems, some of which may be the same as, or at least
similar to, your own. Learning how other people cope can be a tremendous
source of support, especially if you really want to cope better but are not
always sure how to do it.

Support groups can also be wonderful for your family, giving spouses,
partners, children, parents, and others the chance to get some support of
their own. And since one of the most important factors in handling is having a supportive family behind you, you should most certainly encourage
their participation.

Groups that are run by professional leaders or facilitators can be helpful to those with OA. These groups are great places to share your feelings
and gain valuable information and strategies in a constructive, therapeutically beneficial way. Remember that groups are not designed to give false
hope. They are meant to enable you to express and share real feelings, to
learn real strategies, and to derive hope from individuals living in similar
circumstances.

In groups, any topics you'd like to talk about can be discussed. You
may begin to share feelings more openly when you hear others talking
about subjects you were previously reluctant to bring up yourself. As a result, a feeling of closeness—almost a family feeling—will develop.

Sometimes, members of groups dealing with chronic medical conditions discuss feelings of hostility toward the medical profession. Someone
experiencing these feelings may have a hard time communicating with
and trusting physicians. In a group, hopefully, these feelings can be cor-
rected so that a more positive, constructive relationship can be formed
with medical professionals. (Chapter 23 contains more information on improving doctor-patient relationships.)

Don't feel that you *must* be in a group, however. If you're uncomfortable with the idea, or you really don't think it's necessary because you're

involved in other support activities, that's okay. Just make sure that you're honest with yourself. Don't feel that you have to share your emotional reactions with others. It's not necessary to talk them out, despite the potential benefits. But do realize that these emotions need to be recognized and worked through. That's the only way to make progress.

You can obtain information about locating a support group from your local chapter of the Arthritis Foundation. It may also be worthwhile to contact sources such as local hospitals, your physician or other health-care providers, the state medical society, local schools of psychology or social work, religious organizations, libraries, and the Internet. Or you can always start a group of your own.

The Arthritis Foundation offers services to individuals and family members living with this condition. Regardless of whether or not you participate in a support group, it can be beneficial to join this organization, receive materials from them, and learn additional ways that they can be of help.

EXPLORE PROFESSIONAL COUNSELING

Professional counseling can help whenever some aspect of your life becomes overwhelming, your emotional problems become severe, or you want to prevent problems from getting worse. Certainly, any period of change can be made easier with the help of a support professional such as a psychologist, psychiatrist, social worker, psychiatric nurse, pastoral counselor, or another professional with the necessary credentials, compassion, and expertise.

Having somebody to talk to can be a big help. The occasions when you speak to your counselor may be among the few times when you can be totally honest, and at the same time get feedback that can help you better deal with your feelings. Yes, it can be helpful to talk to family and friends and to other people in your situation. And certainly not everyone needs professional help. But a professional therapist or counselor can provide a kind of frank intervention you can't get anywhere else.

If you don't know of an appropriate professional, you should be able to get a referral from any of the physicians who are treating you, from your local chapter of the OA Association, or from a local hospital or professional organization.

USE EFFECTIVE COPING STRATEGIES

There are a number of coping strategies you can use to better manage the emotions that may be troubling you as you deal with OA. Any of these strategies can help you feel more in control and less depressed.

Make a conscious, constructive agreement with yourself. Tell yourself that you're going to set aside a little time each day to work on strengthening your emotional self and preparing yourself for the next day. During this special time, include activities such as relaxation, imagery, meditation, reading, goal setting, or positive thinking to improve your attitude. By consciously devoting time to this, you not only will improve your overall emotional state, but you also will increase your feelings of control because you're doing something to help yourself.

Let's discuss some of the best techniques you can use to improve the way you feel.

Develop a Positive Mental Attitude

It is so important to have a positive mental attitude. Individuals with good mental attitudes are much better able to take control of their emotions. A negative mental attitude may exacerbate any emotional problems you may experience. So your primary goal should be to do all you can to improve your attitude so that you can improve every other aspect of your life. Many of the strategies you'll learn in this section of the book will help you to improve your attitude.

Books may be very helpful in your efforts to generate a more positive mental outlook. Many offer excellent suggestions. Look into some of these. If you get just one good idea out of a 300-page book, the effort will be worthwhile. (See For Further Reading at the back of this book for some suggestions.)

You want to do whatever you can to emphasize the positive in your life. Improving your attitude is a very important part of that. If you think positive thoughts, you'll feel better, regardless of what's going on around you.

Isn't that worth the effort? Believe it or not, the very act of *seeming* cheerful often leads to feeling this way. So walk tall and hold your head high. Feel good about who you are.

Laugh a Little

Laughter is one of the most effective coping strategies there is. Research has shown that chemicals called endorphins—our body's own natural painkillers—are released by the brain whenever we laugh. These endorphins can block pain and give us a feeling of well-being. Haven't you felt better and experienced a greater sense of well-being after having a good laugh? You can enhance the process of getting and staying better by developing your sense of humor and making laughter an important part of your treatment program.

Humor is a pleasurable and effective way to deal with emotions. Whether you're listening to someone else's joke, laughing at yourself, or telling your own joke, humor can be a big help in troublesome situations. Although there isn't much that's funny about having OA, it helps to look on the bright side and lighten up a bit.

Humor works in three ways. First of all, it reduces anxiety. Laughter is one of the best ways known to release tension. This is important because tension exacerbates pain, while relaxation reduces it.

Second, laughter can distract you from those feelings or thoughts that are bothering you. When you're involved in something humorous, you often feel a lot better. Think back, for example, to a time when you were depressed or uncomfortable, and somebody asked if you had heard a certain joke. Initially, you might have been reluctant to hear it. But before long, you were probably totally absorbed in the joke, wondering what the punch line would be. The fact that humor can distract you also means that it can help you see things from a different perspective. So you may be able to look at something more objectively, which can help you handle it more effectively.

Finally, the ability to laugh at yourself is a helpful coping strategy. The degree to which this works, however, depends on what you're going through. It's just about impossible to laugh at yourself while you're initially going through this crisis. However, as you adjust to your condition, you will be better able to use humor as a coping strategy.

So make laughter-filled experiences a part of your everyday life. Watch funny shows on television. Borrow humorous videotapes. Listen to comedy tapes. Read the comics. Learn to recognize the amusing absurdities of daily life. Any of these things will help you have fun and feel better. Not only can they give you a quick boost by helping you distance yourself from what may be troubling you, but they can also improve your overall mood and physical well-being.

Set Goals

Goal-setting can be a very good way of coping with your emotions. What types of goals might you set? A good short-term one might be to purchase and read a new book by one of your favorite authors. A long-term goal could involve the planning of a family vacation or activity, or, perhaps, a reunion with out-of-town friends. By setting realistic and positive goals and working to achieve them, you'll be giving yourself pleasurable events to look forward to, and a reason for getting through every day.

Be Nice to Yourself

Because you've been diagnosed with a progressive disease for which there is no cure, you may feel that you've lost some degree of control over your life. You may even feel—incorrectly—that you're being punished. It can be very helpful to offset these feelings by emphasizing the fact that nice things still happen to you. Often, it is important for individuals with chronic medical conditions to be just a little bit more "selfish"—that is, to initiate the kinds of activities or changes that will make them feel better. Of course, this should not be done in a way that is offensive to others. Instead, it should be done in a way that states repeatedly, "I am a worthwhile person, and I deserve to have nice things in my life."

Some people find it very difficult to be nice to themselves. Others may take it to the opposite extreme. They may be so nice to themselves that they have to temper their enthusiasm so as not to become totally self-centered!

What are some of the ways in which you can be nice to yourself? Consider buying yourself little goodies, giving yourself some special time to relax, involving yourself in favorite activities, spending more time with the people you enjoy, and so on. You may want to make a list of those things that would be most interesting and pleasurable for you.

Be Nice to Others

Sometimes one of the best ways to boost your own self-esteem is to be nice to other people. The feeling of pleasure you get from helping others can be very gratifying, and can improve the way you feel about yourself.

What are some of the things you can do to be nice to others? You can help virtually any person in practically any aspect of his or her life, whether at home, work, or play. Visiting people in hospitals, nursing homes, and the like is one way to spread sunshine. Performing voluntary services in such organizations as churches, schools, and civic organizations is another possibility.

Helping others will make you feel better about yourself. Helping others with OA, in particular, can make a big difference in your life. You'll feel more productive. And, perhaps just as helpful, you'll find new ways of reducing boredom and channeling any excess energy or tension.

Derive Comfort from Faith and Spirituality

Individuals with strong religious faith often derive a tremendous amount of solace from prayer and focus on matters beyond everyday concerns. The religious beliefs of family and friends can also be a source of comfort to both you and them. Of course, the way in which you nourish your spiritual side is up to you. Don't feel that you have to turn to any particular type of practice if it does not seem natural to you, but do try to be aware of all aspects and levels of your experience.

Make Use of Relaxation Techniques

Relaxation is the opposite of tension. Therefore, if you learn to relax, you'll be much less tense. Moreover, tension exacerbates pain, whereas relaxation reduces it.

Relaxation procedures by themselves will not totally control your emotions. But if you're feeling more relaxed, you'll be better able to identify those problems affecting you, and then be better able to deal with them. So relaxation procedures can be an essential first step in coping with your emotions.

How can you relax? We're talking about clinical relaxation now—not everyday activities like reading, gardening, listening to music, or sitting in front of the television with a bowl of popcorn! There are several different types of clinical relaxation procedures, including progressive relaxation, meditation, autogenics, deep breathing, and a technique called the quick release. Imagery, hypnosis, and biofeedback are three techniques that can be used for a number of different purposes, including relaxation. (See Chapter 5.)

Remember that if you have difficulty learning to relax on your own, there is nothing wrong with working with a professional who can help you learn these skills.

Pinpoint What's Bothering You

Are you more comfortable now? Then you're ready to proceed to the next crucial step. In order to deal with anything that's upsetting you, you have to determine exactly what it is that's bothering you. Make a list of these things. Then go over what you've written. In reviewing your list, you'll see that just about every item can be placed in one of two categories. The first category contains the "modifiables"—the problems or emotions that you can do something about. The second category includes the "nonmodifiables"—the things you can't do anything about. Why separate them? Because different strategies should be used to deal with each of these two types of problems.

For the first category, you'll want to figure out what techniques you can use to improve the situation. As for the second category, you'll still be planning strategies, but of a different kind.

Where do your emotions exist? In your mind, right? Therefore, your plan for this category is to work on the way you're thinking.

Work on Your Thinking

How can you change your thinking so that something will bother you less? The technique you choose should depend on the specific emotional reaction that's bothering you. For example, if you're afraid of something and you want to conquer this fear, a procedure called systematic desensitization may be helpful. (We'll go into this in Chapter 15.) Then again, if you're feeling guilty or angry about something, or if something is depressing you, it can be very helpful to learn how to change or "restructure" the way you're thinking. (You'll learn more about techniques for this in Chapters 14, 16, and 17.)

How do you deal with uncertainty? One of the first things to do is to focus on living as a person who happens to have OA, rather than seeing yourself as a victim of OA. Try to live life fully and enjoy it as much as possible. And try to live as normally as possible. Concentrate on what you have, rather than dwelling on things you don't have. Concentrate on what you can do each day, not what you can no longer do. Those who are successful live one day at a time, making the most of each day.

Actually, any of the techniques we've discussed can be used to cope with just about any problem. It's simply a question of deciding what works best for you.

LOOKING TOWARD THE FUTURE

You are the same person you were before you developed OA. The fact that you have it doesn't mean that anything else about you has changed. Keep this in mind, and try to maintain as much control over your life as you can. If there are ways in which you can improve your control, do so.

If you find yourself experiencing intense emotional reactions, have faith that these feelings will diminish, either due to the passage of time or because of something you do to help yourself. You can expect to experience more emotional reactions during those times when your symptoms are more pronounced. But even when these feelings do occur, you should be able to point to so many positive things in your life that it may be easier to deal with these feelings. In this way, you'll be able to develop the positive mental attitude that you want to become an integral part of your life.

The purpose of the following seven chapters is to help you to understand different emotions you may be experiencing. You'll discover where these emotions come from, and recognize that many other individuals have gone through exactly what you're going through now. In addition, a number of strategies will be presented to help you cope with these emotions more effectively. Remember that "practice makes better." Just reading about a method used to control an emotion doesn't guarantee success. You have to keep on practicing. So don't be afraid, depressed, angry, or guilty. Instead, read on!

CHAPTER THIRTEEN

Coping with the Diagnosis

When you first found out you had osteoarthritis, how did you feel? How did you react when your doctor gave a name to your pain? People with OA may experience a whole range of emotions when they are diagnosed. These emotions may include anger, fear, and feelings of being out of control. Some people cry. Some feel frustration. Others feel numb.

Many people with OA, especially with primary OA, aren't terribly surprised. They may have expected that there be some medical explanation for their joints' hurting more and more. Now at least the disease has a name and treatment can begin. People with secondary osteoarthritis may not take the diagnosis as well, because they may not have been expecting it, and they may see it as interfering more drastically with their lifestyle. For example, an athlete who develops secondary osteoarthritis may fear a premature end to his or her career.

Some of the more common reactions to a diagnosis of OA, such as anxiety, relief, and denial will be discussed in this chapter.

Initial Reactions

Let's look in greater detail at some of the more common reactions to diagnosis. Later on in the chapter, we'll look at how you can begin to cope with these emotions.

ANXIETY

What might you be thinking at the time of diagnosis? Immediately after diagnosis, a commonly experienced reaction—and certainly not a pleasant one—is anxiety. Regardless of how long your symptoms have taken to develop, you might be thinking, "Oh, no, I have OA! What's going to happen to me? Am I going to end up needing a wheelchair?" Or you may say, "I don't want an 'old-age' disease. I'm too young for this!" Or you may ask, "Will I ever get better?" "What is the treatment—and how will I handle it?" "Who will take care of me?" You may believe that your life will never be the same again. Family members and loved ones may have similar fears and questions. They may feel anxious as well as helpless, because they don't know what they can do for you. This can certainly make things worse—for them *and* for you.

Let's talk about this reaction. It's normal to be upset and afraid. Does anyone you know like pain or physical restrictions? Of course not. You may suddenly be hit with the fact that you are mortal and vulnerable. You'll realize you may have this problem for the rest of your life. Physically, it's not uncommon to feel faint or dizzy, or to experience other stress reactions at the time of diagnosis.

Although it may take time to come to terms with the diagnosis, the process of acceptance began the moment you heard the diagnosis. And acceptance must take place. It is an important step in learning to deal with your condition.

RELIEF

Does everyone feel anxious and afraid when diagnosed? Not at all. Some people actually feel relieved! Why? Perhaps you were experiencing a lot of pain and nothing seemed to help. Maybe your family and friends thought you were the pain was more in your head than in your joints. Maybe you thought you might have a tumor or a life-threatening illness that was causing the pain, and were relieved to find out that wasn't the case.

There are other reasons you might be relieved after your diagnosis. First, you're probably hopeful that treatment will significantly improve the way you've been feeling (and it's good to finally know *why* you're feeling that way). Second, family members and friends who may have thought you were exaggerating your symptoms or, possibly, didn't even believe that you were really in pain will now discover you were telling the truth. Third, and most important, you'll be relieved that *it wasn't all in your head.* After a long period of time, even the most confident person can begin to wonder if there is really something wrong or if the problem is purely psychological.

The Process of Adjusting

You and your family will probably experience a number of major emotional reactions as you adjust to the idea of having OA. Later on in this section of the book, there are complete chapters devoted to depression, fear, anger, and guilt. But what about the other emotions? Let's take a brief look at some other feelings and reactions you may experience during your adjustment period.

DENIAL

It may be difficult for you to accept the fact that you have OA. Regardless of what symptoms you've been experiencing, you may go through a period of denial. That is, you might be willing to deal with the symptoms, but not with having a permanent label attached to them. So you may protest, "Oh, come on, I've just been overdoing things lately. I don't have a *disease*"; "If

I give it a little time, I'm sure the problem will go away by itself"; or even "#*$&x%!!—leave me alone!"

Did you ever ask yourself, "Why can't things go back to the way they used to be?" Have you ever wished you could wake up one morning and find out that this was a bad dream? The more you keep hoping that it will go away, the more you are slowing down your adjustment. Why is this so? Because you're not really admitting to yourself that you have changed— perhaps permanently. Such denial can make it harder to cope with having OA, since you are not facing the problem realistically.

Believe it or not, though, there are times when denial can be positive. How? By keeping you from dwelling on problems when that won't make them any better. In other words, if there's nothing you can do to improve a situation, why keep thinking about it? Remember that although denial does distort reality, there may be times when distortion is necessary. So denial can be helpful early on, following diagnosis, as you get used to dealing with that diagnosis. It may enable you to go about your normal routine while you're getting used to these unpleasant circumstances. But as time goes by, denial can go from being appropriate to being inappropriate if it keeps you from doing what you have to do in order to help yourself. Family members may also be in denial. But when they allow denial to continue, they may be unknowingly contributing to your inappropriate way of dealing with the problem.

If you're reading this book, then chances are you're probably not denying your OA. But if you *are* denying it, the best way to start coping with your situation is to face reality. Speak to those professionals who know about your condition, and have them explain it in further detail. Let them explain why treatment is necessary. Look at any x-rays that have been taken. Try to recognize that your condition does exist, that it affects you, and that it will remain with you. Try to plan all your activities and aim all your thinking toward the notion that you are going to do what you can to handle it effectively.

Talk to other people with OA, and listen to what they experienced in the earlier stages of their disease. You will find that many of their stories are similar to your own. You may also discover self-help groups that can add to your knowledge of OA, as well as your coping ability.

UNCERTAINTY

There is always uncertainty in our lives. Now you're faced with a new un-certainty—uncertainty regarding OA treatment, outcome, symptoms, your ability to pursue your work and life goals, and so on.

Even if treatment is successful, there can still be uncertainty as to fu-ture problems. The important thing is to focus on the certainties in your life. Do as many things normally as you can. Don't play the role of a sick person. Get on with the act of living.

DAMAGED SELF-ESTEEM

One of the most important characteristics that each of us has is our self-esteem. The way you feel about yourself is very important and helps you get through each day. Unfortunately, OA can have a damaging effect on self-esteem. Feelings of confidence can be quickly shattered, and this can have a very unpleasant effect. You may not feel or behave like yourself. You'll want to deal with this right away in order to return to effective, effi-cient functioning.

One problem that can affect your self-esteem is the feeling that you're no longer independent and that you've lost a certain amount of control over your life. For example, you may feel there is little you can do about the pain. The degree to which this feeling exists varies from person to per-son. Medical visits, surgery, medication, treatments, waiting to hear from others about "the next step"—all these things make you more dependent on the medical system. And this may continue for the rest of your life. If you allow it, your self-esteem may suffer because you feel more dependent on others, particularly in your dealings with the health-care system or in the hospital, where others control virtually every aspect of your life.

What can you do about this? Instead of being upset by the things you can't do or the ways in which you are dependent on others, focus on the things you *can* do! Try to maintain as normal a routine as you can. Take control over as much of your life as possible. Get involved in support groups. Speak to others to find out how they handle these very important issues. If necessary, speak to a professional counselor.

In addition, changes in body image can occur as a result of OA. For example, you may develop Heberden's or Bouchard's nodes and feel uncomfortable about your appearance because of that. You may not like the way you look. This can change the way you feel about your body, and can have a very profound effect on your self-esteem.

What can you do to improve your body image? One approach is to look for ways to enhance your appearance. For instance, you might consider wearing clothing designed to refocus the attention of others away from certain parts of your body. If you are overweight, consider following a dietary program to lose weight. But remember that many body changes are *internal*, and aren't noticeable to others. So the most significant step you can take may be to work on your attitude. Remind yourself of who you are, and who you've always been. Feel good about the things that are truly important, and minimize the rest.

NEGATIVE THOUGHTS

It is important to push away negative thoughts. For example, some people blame themselves for their illness—or feel that they're being punished for something they did. This type of thinking doesn't do any good; in fact, it can be counterproductive. Everyone has negative thoughts—thoughts that lead to the growth and intensity of negative emotions. However, there is no law that says you have to let these thoughts continue. Keep challenging these thoughts. Work to turn them around and make them more rational, realistic, and positive. In this way, you'll continue to focus on the positive feelings that are such an essential part of successfully living with OA.

It is a waste of valuable energy to be angry, guilt-ridden, self-blaming, or self-critical. It's now time to harness the energy that goes into these negative emotions, and to turn it into positive energy that can strengthen you.

How Can You Begin to Adjust?

You may have many questions immediately following your diagnosis. Regardless of the way you reacted to your diagnosis, OA is not something that can be ignored. It is just as important to be able to handle your emotions as it is to handle the medical aspects of the disease. It's important to understand the condition, cope with it, and incorporate it into your life. You want to fit OA into your life—not change your life to fit OA, although sometimes you may find yourself doing just this! The most important question is one that only you can answer: "Will I give up living because of OA, or will I continue to live despite OA?" The following steps should start you on the path to living successfully with OA.

TAKE CHARGE

You must take the reins and begin to help yourself. Sure, you can receive love and support from your family and friends, and obtain guidance and expertise from professionals. But that's not enough. You are the one who is going to have to come to grips with OA. At first, adjusting may be difficult. But there is no other way out. You must face it. As you do, it is important to have a sense of empowerment—to be in control of as many factors in your life as possible.

Even if your initial reaction to the diagnosis of OA is negative, this will pass. Later on, your disease may cause new or stronger symptoms. You may have been going along after treatment, feeling pretty good. And then—wham—you get hit with a new set of problems. If this happens, face it, take charge, and use the techniques presented here to help you once again.

INFORMATION, PLEASE!

Many of your initial reactions were probably the result of not knowing enough about OA. So you'll want to learn as much as possible. Your physician should be helpful in suggesting ways of getting current information.

It's very easy to let your imagination run wild. Initially, you'll probably keep thinking about all the things that can possibly go wrong. You'll worry about every symptom. You may also become frightened about OA affecting more joints than it currently does, as well as how it might affect you and the people close to you. So learn the facts about your condition. This is a great way to alleviate some of the anxiety caused by the diagnosis.

After reading current, general, consumer-oriented information, you might want to move on to more technical material. Ask your doctor about anything you don't understand. And certainly ask questions about anything that frightens you. After all, medical writing is not designed to calm the person with OA. It merely states medical facts and statistics. Don't forget this, or you may become unnecessarily alarmed.

It probably wasn't a lifelong goal of yours to become an expert on OA, but think about how much this information may help you. Doctors will respect your questions more. And you'll understand exactly what's going on in your body. These are just two of the many advantages that can come from reading about your condition.

Should you believe everything you read? Of course not. You may come across any number of miracle "cures" and alternative treatments advertised in newspapers and magazines or on the Internet. Other people who find out about your diagnosis may send you information about OA and its treatment, or try to share stories about others with OA. Make sure that whatever you read comes from a reputable source, and remember that it takes rigorous scientific study before one can prove that a new procedure or treatment is actually effective. And be sensible. If some exciting new treatment or medication were discovered, wouldn't you expect to learn about it in your daily newspaper or on a national news program? Things that sound too good to be true almost always are.

Many valuable facts about OA can be obtained from the Arthritis Foundation. Don't hesitate to call them and tell them the kind of information you're looking for so that they can provide you with helpful materials. These and other groups may be located in your area, or they may have national offices that can provide you with up-to-date information. (See the Resource Groups section for further details.)

You can also obtain a lot of information online. There are dozens of reputable, beneficial web sites about OA (some of these are listed in the Resource Groups section).

BEGIN FACING YOUR FEARS

Once you've accepted the fact that you have OA, you can start determining what changes you may have to make in your lifestyle. In addition, you will want to try to control as many harmful emotions as you can.

The emotions stemming from the diagnosis of OA can be unpleasant. You may experience regret, sorrow, nostalgia, and anger, remembering the way life used to be. Many fears may come to mind, some of which may be overwhelming. Fears of incapacitation, of surgery, and of losing out on life are all very common. Begin facing them. They can and must be faced in order to move your adjustment along more smoothly.

DEVELOP A POSITIVE RELATIONSHIP WITH YOUR DOCTOR

Obviously, you must work with a physician you can trust, one who has had experience working with people with OA. You want to learn as much as possible about the different treatments for OA. And you can start by asking questions of your physician. Remember that the patient-physician relationship is very important when dealing with any chronic illness. If your physician does not seem receptive to your questions, try to make him aware of how important these questions are to you. If no progress is made, then you may have to reconsider this relationship and look for another doctor. (More on working with your physician in Chapter 23.)

HELP YOUR FAMILY ADJUST

The processing of adjusting to the diagnosis of OA can be harder if the people close to you also have difficulty with their emotions—especially if their emotions are different from yours.

Loretta, a fifty-six-year-old receptionist, had only recently been diagnosed as having OA. After a few depressing weeks, however, she began to learn how to cope. She was finally able to handle thoughts of future lifestyle changes, concerns about reduced mobility, and some of the other unpleasant thoughts associated with OA. Sound great? Not really. You see, her husband of thirty-seven years was resentful that his wife had a progressive disease that made her unable to do everything she used to do, her children were worried that she was going to become dependent on them, and her mother was feeling guilty because, at eighty-two, she was quite healthy. Although Loretta was learning how to cope with OA, she could not cope with her family. They were making things very difficult for her.

When any member of the family has a health problem, it has an effect on other family members. They, too, will go through periods of denial—times at which they'll say, "I'm sure the problem will clear up by itself," or, perhaps, hint that you might be exaggerating the degree of your symptoms and their impact on your life. Unfortunately, this won't make things easier for you. If family members seem to be having problems related to your illness, it is a good idea for them to seek out people to speak to—just as it may benefit *you* to seek help. Spouses, children, and others can find out more about OA and learn how others cope with treatment. They can even join support groups or seek counseling. Encourage your family members and to learn as much as they can and to seek whatever help they need. Their adjustment will help your adjustment.

ADD TO YOUR SUPPORT SYSTEM

The time when you're diagnosed with OA is not a time to be alone. It's a time to reach out—to get support from family and friends whom you value. In addition, support groups, the Arthritis Foundation, and your doctor may be able to help you make contact with other people with OA in your area so you can talk to them and learn as much as you can from people who have "been there."

In Closing

Start thinking positively about your life with OA. Learn as much as you can about your condition. Use whatever support systems are necessary. Use all the stress-management and emotion-control techniques you can learn. (Many good ones can be found in this book.) Start saying to yourself, "OA may be affecting me, but I'm going to adjust and live a long, fulfilling life."

If it's necessary for you to make changes in your lifestyle—even major ones—tell yourself that you will make them, and that you will make them willingly. You're going to lead as complete a life as you can. The more quickly you can adjust your lifestyle to fit your needs, the more rapidly you'll be able to enjoy your life. You are not helpless, and you can make the most of your life despite OA!

CHAPTER FOURTEEN

Depression

Sam was a 64-year old man who had been married for forty-four years, and he and his wife had successfully raised three children. They now lived in a beautiful home in a well-to-do neighborhood. It looked as though he had everything anyone could ask for. But he hadn't asked for OA! And oh, what an effect this had on him! In the past, Sam had always been enthusiastic about life. But he now became extremely unhappy whenever he thought about the future. He felt that he couldn't get around the way he used to, and was afraid he would end up needing a wheelchair. He didn't even want to spend time with his children or grandchildren. Sam was suffering from depression.

Depression is a serious problem. Although actual numbers vary, it is estimated that at least 5 million Americans require professional care for depression. Because it is so widespread, depression has been nicknamed the "common cold" of emotional problems.

Just what is depression? Depression is an extremely unpleasant, persistent feeling of unhappiness and despair. It can range from a mild problem—feeling discouraged and downhearted—to a severe disorder—feeling utterly hopeless, worthless, and unwilling to go on living. You may feel that there is no reason to remain a part of the world. You may be afraid of being a burden to your family, and think that everybody would be better off without you. Or you may just feel useless.

Depression can be painful. Imagine how it must hurt to feel (or say), "I wish I were never born. What good am I? I'm not helping anybody around me, and I'm not helping myself." It may seem as if the whole world is against you. Life may seem unfair—a constant struggle in which you never win. And that hurts.

What Are the Symptoms of Depression?

There are a number of possible symptoms of depression. If you notice that you're feeling excessive amounts of sadness, despair, discouragement, or melancholy; if you're unable to eat; if you're sleeping either too much or too little; if you feel totally withdrawn from social activities; if you find yourself crying often, and that's not typical behavior for you; if you're brooding about the past and feeling hopeless—any of these feelings may indicate depression. And there are other symptoms, as well. If you're excessively irritable or angry; if your fears seem to be extreme; if you feel inadequate and worthless; if you are unable to concentrate on virtually anything in your life, whether it be work, family, or other interests; if you seem to have little or no interest in activities that previously gave you pleasure; if you have reduced amounts of energy that don't seem to be related to the disease or treatment; if you have little or no interest in sex or intimacy; and if your cognitive style (the way you speak, think, and act) seems to be generally slowing down—these, too, can be symptomatic of depression. You may have difficulty concentrating, and your attention span may be much shorter. When you speak (and you'll probably do less of that, too), your conversation will usually be shallow, emphasizing feelings of worthlessness and despair. The more of these symptoms you experience, the more likely it is that you are depressed and should take some action to help yourself.

HOW DEPRESSION AFFECTS YOUR BODY

Some of the more noticeable symptoms of depression are physical in nature, such as nervous activity or agitation or wringing of the hands. You may be restless or have difficulty remaining in one place. On the other hand, you may become much less active and remain motionless for abnormally long periods of time—even appearing as if you are in a trance, with no apparent desire to do anything. Sam's wife, Helen, became very concerned when her husband remained seated in a chair in the living room for hours at a time. When she asked him a question, he would respond in monosyllables. When friends called on the phone, he never wanted to talk to them. Sam's depression was causing him to lose interest in just about everything.

If you're depressed, most of your physical activities will also slow down—and not just because of any physical limitations due to OA. You're probably feeling exhausted. This may be surprising, since you're not doing much of anything. But constantly telling yourself that you're no good can be tiring in itself! You really don't want to believe this, but you feel as if you have no choice. And in attempting to escape from these feelings, you may become even more depressed—as well as more physically drained and exhausted.

Depression may also cause you to feel physically sick or to experience a change in appetite. Of course, it's wise to remember that any of these symptoms might be related to OA or another physical disorder. So even if the symptoms go away once your depression improves, don't just assume that they're related only to the depression. A thorough medical examination may still be a good idea. This way, you'll be sure that there is no organic cause for your depression.

HOW DEPRESSION AFFECTS YOUR MOODS AND OUTLOOK

If you're depressed, you may experience frequent mood swings. For example, you might feel worse in the morning and better in the evening. This may be because of depression as well as the joint stiffness and pain of OA. And any nightly improvement may occur because each evening you realize that it's almost time to go to sleep—to escape. But depression may also make sleep difficult, even if you weren't doing much of anything during the day. If you're mildly depressed, you may have difficulty concentrating, and your attention span may be much shorter. When you speak, your conversation may suggest, or even express, feelings of worthlessness and despair.

When you're depressed, it feels as if your mood keeps getting lower. You like yourself very little, if at all. Your thinking is very negative and very different from the way it was when you were feeling good. In fact, it is this negative thinking—not just a particular triggering event—that leads to depression in the first place. (More on this later in the chapter.)

Your day-to-day activities may suffer as a result of these negative feelings. You may, for instance, spend the day in your bathrobe simply because you don't feel like dressing. Or you may go through the motions of your everyday activities, even though your heart isn't in them. Many people, in fact, simply withdraw from their usual activities during bouts of depression. Some people even find themselves wishing they could die rather than having to go through the pain and disability their OA is causing. They feel their joints are only going to deteriorate more, the pain is only going to get worse, and there will be more and more things they can't do, so why bother living? If you've ever felt this way, don't feel guilty about such thoughts. You're not alone. But you should take these feelings seriously and, if necessary, see a mental health professional. These feelings can and will go away if you work hard enough on them.

HOW DEPRESSION AFFECTS YOUR RELATIONSHIPS

If you're depressed, you may feel that people around you have no need for you. As Sam used to complain, "Why should my friends want to see me or make plans with me? I can't do anything!"

Do you feel less at ease talking to others than you used to? Does it seem as if others are having a hard time talking to you, even if they have been close to you for a long time? As already discussed, due to your depression, you may be less interested in conversation and you may feel less confident. You may project your negative feelings about yourself onto others, and believe that they really don't want to talk to you. And the more depressed you become, the better you may get at convincing those around you that you're no good. You may feel that others have no need for you. You may think that they consider you to be an uninteresting, boring person.

Ann received a telephone call from her friend Regina. Regina wanted to know how Ann had been feeling, since the last time they had gotten together Ann had seemed to be in a great deal of pain. Ann responded half-heartedly, imagining that Regina was calling only out of obligation. She then explained that she would understand if Regina did not want to call again, since she never seemed to have any good news to tell her. How do you think Regina felt? Imagine hearing this repeatedly, despite having reassured Ann that her concern was sincere. Would you be surprised if, eventually, Regina got tired of even trying, and simply stopped calling? But in Ann's mind, this would only reinforce her feelings that she really was no good—that she was not worthy of having any friends after all.

What Causes Depression?

A bout of depression frequently starts with one specific thing—one upsetting event or occurrence. Lenny had been planning a holiday cruise with his family for more than a year. Although he had been in more pain recently, he was still looking forward to the cruise. In the weeks prior to the trip, however, Lenny was experiencing so much pain that his doctor advised against his going on the trip. This one disappointment triggered a long depression. Lenny felt as if the most important things in his life were being ruined by his OA.

What happens after that first depressing event is a kind of chain reaction. It's almost as if the bottom has dropped out of your world. You may feel that you are less able to control your thinking—although this is not true, as we will see later on in the chapter.

Still, a disappointing or upsetting event doesn't *always* lead to depression. So where does it come from, and why does it sometimes take hold? Sometimes we can figure this out, and sometimes we can't. But before we give up, let's discuss some of the possible causes.

HOW ABOUT THE "NORMAL DOWNS"?

A certain amount of depression is normal in anyone's life. We all experience ups and downs. If we never experienced some of the downs, how could we fully appreciate the ups? However, when depression becomes more than just the "normal downs," it must be addressed. Nipping it quickly in the bud can keep it from becoming much worse.

Of course, certain events—traumatic experiences such as losing a loved one, being diagnosed with a chronic medical problem, requiring major surgery, or being fired from a job—can lead anyone into a depression. However, this doesn't mean that you should ignore the problem or wait until it goes away. It's necessary to learn how to deal with depression. This is an essential part of coping.

HOW ABOUT ANGER YOU CAN'T EXPRESS?

What if you get so angry that you feel like you're going to burst? But you don't—or can't—do anything about it, so you decide to "swallow" your anger. It seems strange that a powerful emotion like anger can turn into a withdrawn, helpless feeling like depression. But it can. If you become increasingly angry about something and feel unable to do anything about it, you may turn that anger inward. You may experience so much frustration or hopelessness that you shut down emotionally in an attempt to keep yourself from experiencing these terrible feelings. This leads to withdrawal, which is one symptom of depression. (More information on anger will be found in Chapter 16.)

COULD IT BE A CHEMICAL IMBALANCE?

In a small percentage of cases, depression may be caused by biochemical imbalances in the body. However, this does not occur very often. Treatment for biochemical depression may involve the use of drugs in an effort to rebalance body chemistry. But this usually isn't the whole answer. Regardless of whether your depression is caused by this or, more typically, by your reactions to the people and events around you, you should try to modify your behavior and improve your thinking. Many experts believe that even if the cause of depression is biochemical, by working on the way you handle your day-to-day living, you can have a positive effect on your mood.

CAN OA ITSELF CAUSE DEPRESSION?

Can OA cause depression? Are you kidding? The pain and other symptoms of this disease can certainly either create or magnify already existing depression. Depression sometimes starts even before diagnosis—especially if you've gotten fed up with your pain—and can reappear periodically during your life with the disease. This is normal, and is something you'll want to work on to minimize the frequency and length of the episodes.

One contributor to depression in people with OA is frustration in their need for control. Most people have the need to feel they have mastery over at least certain aspects of their lives, and OA may make you feel that you've lost control. But even though it may be difficult to admit to yourself that you may not be in control of everything, remind yourself that you can still control certain things. It's much better to focus your energy in this direction.

You may also experience a feeling of helplessness. You may feel weak, uncertain about the future, and powerless to help yourself. This can certainly lead to depression.

What else about OA may depress you? You may become depressed thinking about the future, wondering how OA will affect your life. Knowing that you need (or may need) support devices can be depressing, as well as the fact that you'll probably need medication to deal with the pain. Problems involving other people may depress you, too. For example, you could feel helpless at not being able to share what you're experiencing and be depressed that others can't relate to what you're going through. People may expect more from you than you are able or willing to do. You may be depressed over the possibility of damaged relationships or family friction.

If you're single, you may be heartbroken at the thought that OA will affect possible future relationships—not that there need be any truth to this at all.

Depression may also result from lifestyle changes. What if you are not able to participate in all of the activities you used to love? What if you have to change your work routine, as well as your family routine? What if you experience money problems? Any of these issues can certainly be depressing. Just having OA, with its effects on your day-to-day living, can get to you.

You may be saying to yourself, "If I'm depressed over my OA, how can I expect to get over it unless my OA is cured?" This kind of thinking will get you nowhere. You don't want your emotional state to depend on your physical state. So if your depression lingers, don't wait. Work on it, and learn how to cope. We'll talk more later about how you can improve your thinking.

What Maintains Depression?

If you're depressed, you may be blaming yourself—or your OA—for everything that is wrong in your life. You may tend to become more and more withdrawn, and pull away from the world around you. Realistically, withdrawing won't solve anything. But you may feel that it is the only way to stop feeling terrible. Unfortunately, this will only keep you depressed. (In fact, it may make you even more depressed than you are already.)

Although you may seem sullen and withdrawn to others, you're probably in deep emotional pain. Part of what is making you, and keeping you, depressed is your effort to protect yourself from this emotional pain. You feel that nothing good can possibly happen—that only bad things can happen. So what do you do? You try to block everything out of your mind!

So why do you stay depressed? Why doesn't it just go away? It may be because you don't want to talk to anybody, or even consider counseling. Therefore, the thoughts and feelings that lead to your depression are kept inside. You may ask, "Is my unwillingness to talk the only reason I'm still depressed? If I start talking more, will that get me out of my depression?"

Not necessarily. But it can certainly be helpful to talk out your feelings. It would probably be beneficial if a close friend or family member took the initiative and forced you into some kind of conversation—therapeutic or otherwise—or, at least, pushed you into doing something constructive.

How Can You Cope with Depression?

Can anything be done to end depression? Of course! First, tell yourself that the main reason you're depressed is that you haven't yet taken the proper steps toward feeling better. These steps can pull you out of your rut and reacquaint you with the more positive, pleasant aspects of living—the aspects that you'd like to experience.

Don't think it will be easy, though. Unfortunately, once you've fallen into depression, it takes a certain amount of hard work and persistence to pull yourself out. The result, however, is surely worth the effort. And, of course, it will be easier if you know and use specific techniques and activities that will help. The strategies and techniques that work best to deal with depression can also help to prevent it. Unfortunately, this doesn't mean that you will never become depressed again. It may happen. But if it does, you will be able to recognize it for what it is, and you won't completely fall apart. And if this feeling does come back, won't it be good to know that you *can* do something to help yourself?

One of the first things you must do in learning to cope with depression is to accept any limitations in your life. Admit that you can't control or become involved in *everything*. This doesn't mean that you are powerless, but it does mean that you may have to alter your views about what you can and cannot do. Once you accept your limitations, you will be able to focus your energy in appropriate, constructive directions instead of lamenting what has changed. How can you accept your limitations? Well, let's say that you were previously able to do twenty-five things in your life and now, because of OA, you are unable to do ten of those things. Instead of wasting your energy thinking about the things you can no longer do, focus your energy on feeling good about the ones you can do! Remember the Serenity Prayer: "Grant me the serenity to accept the things I cannot change, the courage to change the things I can, and the wisdom to know the difference."

Regardless of what you have to do and what mountains seem to stand in your way, the most you can ask of yourself—the most that anybody can ask—is to take one step at a time. Just keep taking one more step. This will be helpful, especially if you're feeling a little overwhelmed.

Now that you're ready to fight your depression, consider two major ways of dealing with it: being more physical (in other words, doing something), and working on your thinking. It can be very helpful to make a list of all the things that are depressing you. You may feel there will be at least fifty items. But in actuality, you'll probably start running out of ideas after six or seven. Next, divide this list into two more lists: first, those things that you can do something about, and, second, those things you can't do anything about. So get physical and do something about those items in the first list, and get thoughtful—work on your thinking—regarding those items in the second list.

LET'S GET PHYSICAL

There are two ways of getting physical in order to deal with depression: actively working to accomplish goals, and increasing physical activity. Hopefully, as I've suggested, you've listed all the things that are depressing you, and have made a separate list of those items that can be changed. Now think about ways in which you can modify or eliminate the items on this list. Be realistic but aggressive in planning ways to reach your goals—even if it can't be done all at once.

Where does the physical activity come in? You may unknowingly be using a lot of energy to keep yourself depressed. You may be working hard to keep that anger inside, even if it appears to others that you're simply withdrawing. If your depression is anger turned within, we can logically assume that by releasing your anger, you'll be able to eliminate your feelings of depression. But what should you do with those feelings? You must find an object toward which your anger can be expressed. This may be difficult. However, it's important to release the trapped anger so that it doesn't build up further and deepen your depression.

Think about the following scenario: You're sitting there, depressed and withdrawn. Somebody makes an innocent remark, and you practically bite that person's head off. What's happening? Whatever was said triggered the release of the internalized anger that was making you depressed. Look out, world!

What kinds of activities can help you release your anger? Many physical activities can be effective, depending, of course, on what you're physically able to do. Try walking, playing golf or tennis, or swimming. Yoga, meditation, and exercise classes are great ways to release anger. In addition to being a healthful way of defusing anger, exercise helps to fight depression by encouraging the body to produce *endorphins,* the body's natural "feel-good" substances. Endorphins are neurotransmitters that promote a sense of well-being and can help to give you a more positive attitude. Be sure to get your doctor's okay before beginning any exercise program. This is particularly important if you are over thirty-five and/or have been sedentary for any length of time. (For more information on coping with anger, see Chapter 16. For more information on exercise, see Chapter 9.)

LET'S GET THOUGHTFUL

Although getting physical may help lift your depression—and can also provide a great distraction, which may help you to look at things more objectively—physical activity will not teach you ways of fighting inappropriate thinking. Remember that it's your *thoughts* that have made you depressed. Clearly, restructuring your thinking is a key element in alleviating depression and dealing with any negative emotions.

If you can think yourself into depression, then you can think yourself out of it. How? If you're depressed, you're just talking yourself *down.* All your internal comments—or at least most of them—are probably putdowns: harsh, negative statements that can make you feel even worse. You want your inner voice to help you, not hurt you. Let's see how you can do that.

Distinguish Fact from Fiction

When you're depressed, you tend to distort reality. Clinical research with depressed patients has proven this. Recognize, therefore, that your thoughts are not necessarily based on what is truly happening, but may instead be based on your own distorted views. This is called *cognitive distortion.*

Is this bad? You bet your happiness it is! *Cognitive* refers to your thinking. *Distortion* means you're twisting things around and, in general, losing sight of what's real. We all tend to do this from time to time. But when you're depressed, you do it a lot of the time—if not all of the time—and it keeps you depressed. So how do you stop? First, you must become reacquainted with what is really happening. But how can you do that if you keep distorting reality? Right now, you're better off accepting a trusted friend or family member's perceptions of the situation, because that person is probably a lot more objective and accurate than you are. Since so many feelings of worthlessness are based on distorted facts, depression can be reduced, if not eliminated, once these facts have been straightened out.

Ella kept complaining that none of her friends were calling her. "They don't call as much as they used to. I guess they just don't care." Her daughter, Arlene, asked her to estimate how often her friends used to call. When Ella compared this number to the current number of calls she was receiving, she realized that the numbers were almost the same. She then realized that she was probably just more sensitive than normal. Although she did not feel 100-percent better, Ella did feel a good deal better, because she could now see that she wasn't actually being abandoned.

So make sure you know what's true and what's not. Provide your own assessment of the situation, and be as objective as possible. Then, if necessary, ask other people—people whose opinions you trust—for their evaluation. Work to become more comfortable with any differences in perception and to adjust your thinking so that it more closely resembles the actual circumstances.

Make Molehills Out of Mountains

Does this imply that if you're depressed you have no real problem? Is it "all in your head"? No. Everyone has problems. If you feel good, you can handle them; but if you're depressed, you may feel overwhelmed. And if that happens, each and every unpleasant event or symptom you experience, regardless of how trivial or slight it may be, will tend to depress you.

Again, do your best to view each problem objectively—to avoid blowing it out of proportion. Eventually, as your depression lifts, you will be able to deal with all of life's problems, both big and small.

Avoid Self-Fulfilling Prophecies

We have looked at several thoughts that are characteristic of depression— thoughts that you may be having right now. Are all these thoughts and feelings irrational and untrue? No. But, ironically, although some of them may start off being far from the truth, the longer you feel this way, the greater the chance of their becoming self-fulfilling prophecies. In other words, the more you allow yourself to think negatively, the greater the likelihood that your fears will turn into realities. For example, if you begin telling yourself that friends and relatives don't care, this may become a reality, because your negative attitudes may alienate the people close to you. And if you feel less able or less willing to do the things you used to do, your inactivity is likely to magnify and confirm your feelings of worthlessness, leading to even greater depression and helplessness. Not a pretty picture.

Once you begin feeling depressed, negative thoughts soon lead to negative actions. These negative actions lead to more negative thoughts, which in turn lead to more negative actions, and so on. It is an ongoing vicious cycle that can spiral you further and further downward, into deeper and deeper depression. Eventually you feel trapped in this vicious cycle and believe there's no way to escape.

Are you getting depressed just reading this? In all probability, if you've ever been depressed, you've already said to yourself, "Wow, that sounds just like me!" So if you find that you're starting to believe in your negative thoughts, stop yourself. As I've said before, depression both results from *and* causes a lot of negative thinking. But once you become aware of these thoughts, you can do something about them. People who remain depressed feel incapable of doing anything about their negative thinking, and allow these thoughts to pull them into that vicious cycle mentioned earlier. Try to think positive thoughts, so that if one of your thoughts does turn into a reality, it will at least be a positive one.

Positive Is the Opposite of Negative

How do you stop negative thinking? It may seem that negative thoughts automatically pop into your mind and you cannot stop them. It's like trying to keep your eyes open when you sneeze. You just can't do it. But once you become aware of these thoughts, in fact you *can* do something.

Anna was resting when the telephone rang. "I'm sure that's Kate, calling to cancel our lunch plans," she thought to herself. In the thirty seconds it took her to get to the phone, she became so depressed that she considered not even answering the call. Reluctantly, she answered the phone—and discovered that it was a wrong number! Anna had allowed her negative thoughts to run wild; she had become more and more negative until she was about ready to give up. And for what? There was no real reason for her to think the way she had.

Once she realized that she was thinking this way, what could she have done? She should have *countered* her thoughts. As soon as the thought about Kate calling to cancel entered her mind, she could have told herself, "It may not even be Kate on the phone. Or if it is, maybe she's just calling to confirm. I won't let it bother me now. After all, I don't even know who it is!" Deliberately countering negative thoughts is the beginning of positive thinking.

Dwell on the Brighter Tomorrows

If you find yourself unhappily comparing your present life to life before OA, again, try to modify your thoughts. Start planning fun things for the present and future. Anyone can come up with some enjoyable activities, regardless of his or her physical or financial restrictions. But it takes effort. Refuse to let yourself wallow in self-pity, because that will only allow your depression to overwhelm you. Work on your thinking, develop some positive plans, and translate them into pleasure. Then wave goodbye to your depression!

Of course, if you reflect realistically on your past, you may find that it wasn't much different from the present. You may have had other physical problems. You may have made some mistakes in your life. Naturally, this may make you even more depressed about the future. However, you can't change the past. What's done is done. Keep telling yourself that. Don't punish yourself for the past. Tell yourself that you're going to work on making the future better. Set up some specific goals, starting with the easy-to-reach ones. You'll be helping yourself just by *thinking* about all the positive things you can do!

Rediscover What's Missing from Your Life

You may have laughed when you read the title of this section. "I *know* what's missing from my life—good joints!" you might respond. "Mobility without pain!" Sure. But another important element that might very well be missing—an element that *can* be regained!—is the feeling of satisfaction, accomplishment, and pride that normally comes from others' praise. You may be missing the attention and interest of other people, and this can cause you to feel worthless. What can you do about it? Think about your positive qualities. (Yes, you do have some!) Think about how you can interact more with people, spark their interest, and obtain more of the satisfaction that makes you feel worthwhile.

Shoot for the Earth, Not the Moon

We all have goals for ourselves. It's normal to become depressed when we don't reach a particular one, especially if we've tried very hard to get there. But sometimes our goals are not realistic.

Hal had not returned to work since his hip-replacement surgery. Finally, after a long period of rest and rehabilitation, he was feeling better. His OA was stable, and he was looking forward to getting back to work so that he could catch up on everything. When his doctor finally gave him the go-ahead, he practically flew to his office. After two hours of phone calls, consultations, dictation, and meetings, he was exhausted. His spirits plummeted. He became worried that he'd never again be able to handle all the pressure, and that he was in danger of losing his job. Wrong! Hal had simply set his sights too high. Expecting to return to his old schedule as if he didn't have OA was just not realistic.

Try to judge whether the goals you've been setting for yourself are realistic. If not, reset them, keeping your abilities and limitations in mind. Once your goals are more realistic, you'll have a much better chance of achieving them, and less chance of falling short.

TALK ABOUT IT!

Now you know how to cope with depression both through physical activity and by changing your way of thinking. But there's one more thing you can do—something I've mentioned before. You can *talk* about your problems and concerns with others. Often, the very act of talking will help lift your depression. If you have family members or friends with whom you feel close and whose opinions you trust, approach them. Air your feelings, and listen to their feedback. They may be more objective, and better able to come up with constructive solutions, than you are right now.

If your depression is so intense or prolonged that friends and family are unable to help, then by all means consider speaking to a professional. Counseling is becoming increasingly effective for treating depression. Don't deny yourself this invaluable assistance. Why not do everything you can to help yourself feel better?

An Antidepressing Summary

The best way to work on negative thoughts is to prevent them from continuing. Be realistically positive. Deal with reality the way it actually exists. View thoughts from a more factual point of view. Handle them the way somebody else might—someone who is not depressed and who can be more objective. Try to make your perceptions more accurate, your awareness more realistic, and your thoughts more positive and constructive. Remember: Your thoughts lead to your emotions. If your thoughts are negative and critical, your emotions will be the same. But if you can turn your thoughts around to a more positive, constructive point of view, your emotional reactions will most certainly follow, and depression will be a thing of the past.

CHAPTER FIFTEEN

Fear and Anxiety

Don't be *afraid* to read this chapter! It may help you discover what you're *anxious* about!

The two sentences above may help you distinguish between anxiety and fear. What is the difference? Anxiety is a general sense of uneasiness—a vague feeling of discomfort. It is an agitated, uncertain state in which you just don't feel at peace or in control. There is a premonition that something bad may happen, something that requires protecting yourself. You feel very vulnerable. However, you're not exactly sure about the source of your anxiety.

Fear, on the other hand, is usually more specific. It is often directed toward something that can be recognized, whether a person, an object, a situation, or an event. We may be fearful when we become aware of something dangerous, or when we feel threatened. When we are afraid—much as when we're anxious—we feel out of control and less confident. So the feelings of anxiety and fear are basically the same—the main difference is whether the source of the feeling can be identified. And, most important, the strategies used to combat fear also enable you to cope with anxiety. For this reason, from this point on I will be using the two terms interchangeably.

Fear is so common that we have developed a number of different words to describe it: scared, concerned, alarmed, worried, uptight, nervous, edgy, and shaky. Then there's wary, frightened, and helpless. Is that it? Nope! How about suspicious, hesitant, apprehensive, tense, panicky, disturbed, and agitated? Of course, there are more, but you get the general idea. The important point is that all these words mean the same thing: "I'm afraid." The source of this fear may be either real or imaginary.

What Are the Symptoms of
Fear and Anxiety?

What happens when you become extremely anxious? Your body may react physiologically. You may become short of breath, your heart may beat rapidly, you may feel shaky, and you may think, "I've got to get out of here!" You may attempt to relax but instead stay very tense. You may take a deep breath but find that the breath keeps catching in your throat. You may try to shake the feeling but find that you can't. This inability to calm down can be frightening, and may increase your anxiety even more. A vicious cycle can quickly develop. Before long, you may feel completely out of control.

Which came first, the anxiety or the symptoms? That's really not important. What is more crucial is doing whatever you can to reduce both. That's what will help you to be able to cope with fear—to regain control of your emotions and improve your day-to-day life.

Is Fear Good or Bad?

Believe it or not, fear is usually good! Now, you're probably wondering how this is possible. Fear mobilizes you. It tells you to prepare to attack the source of your fear. You react in a way that leads to action. In this regard, fear is similar to stress. It serves a necessary and critical purpose. In a way, it protects you.

Anxiety is bad only when the source of your fear becomes overlooked, ignored, or denied, or when the feeling is so excessive that it paralyzes you. In such cases, the threat or danger is allowed to continue and nothing—or, at least, not enough—is done to control it.

What Determines the Intensity of Our Reactions?

Fear ranges in intensity from mild to severe. It is impossible to measure just how much fear there is in anyone's life. This varies from person to person and from time to time.

What determines how fearful you get? For one thing, how close is the dreaded object, person, or event? (Wouldn't you be more afraid if you were getting an injection within the next thirty seconds than you would if you were getting one in thirty days?) How vulnerable are you? (Do you truly hate injections, or are you just tired of feeling like a pincushion?) Finally, how successful are you at defending yourself? (Can you calmly accept the needle, or do you scream a lot?) These are just some of the factors that determine how you handle fear.

How Can You Cope with Anxiety and Fear?

Obviously, the more fears you have, the more difficulty you'll experience in making a successful adjustment to your new situation. Recognizing your fears and learning how to deal with them will help you live more happily and comfortably. How? We were afraid you'd never ask! Let's look at some of the ways in which you can help yourself better cope with your fears. Later on in the chapter, we'll look at how you can use some of these strategies—and others, as well—to cope with some specific fears that may be troubling you.

PINPOINT THE SOURCE OF YOUR FEARS

The first step in coping with your fears is to use the pinpointing technique discussed in Chapter 12. Identify and list exactly what scares you and exactly why you are afraid. Then think about what you can do to alleviate your fears.

For Ruth, this was not hard. She knew she was afraid of how people would react when they saw her hands. She quickly realized that what she feared was rejection. She was concerned that they wouldn't want to be with her because of their own fears. ("Could this happen to me?"). She planned a course of action (no, not a one-way ticket to Brazil!). She decided she'd simply do the best she could, expecting her friends to accept her the way she was. If they didn't, that was *their* loss. She was less afraid almost instantly. As you begin planning your strategies and gradually putting your plan into operation, you'll feel better and better.

RELAX!

Because relaxation is the opposite of tension, the use of relaxation techniques can be very helpful in coping with anxieties and fears. As mentioned earlier, there are many types of relaxation techniques: progressive relaxation, meditation, autogenics, deep breathing, and more. Regardless of what is provoking your fear, learning to relax is an important part of improving your emotional well-being. (Detailed information about relaxation techniques can be found in Chapter 5.)

DESENSITIZE YOURSELF

One great technique for conquering fear is called *systematic desensitization.* Using this technique, you gradually desensitize yourself—that is, make yourself less vulnerable and sensitive—to the source of your fear.

Here's how it can work for you. Sit in a comfortable chair and relax. Then create a movie in your mind by imagining whatever it is that makes you afraid. If you get tense, stop imagining it and relax. When you've calmed down, try imagining it again. The more you try to imagine your fear, and alternate this "movie" with relaxation techniques, the less your fears will bother you. Try it! It will give you a great feeling of relaxation and control. There are many books that provide more information on systematic desensitization. Check them out.

LEARN TO COPE WITH ANXIOUS THOUGHTS

As I stated earlier, anxiety is a vague, uneasy feeling with an unknown source. So how can you cope with anxiety by following the steps discussed above? Surely, if you can't pinpoint the source of your fear, you can't follow these specific steps. So what can you do? Well, a number of things may work. Try the relaxation procedures discussed in Chapter 5. Work on changing your thinking to make it more positive and productive. Find somebody to whom you can express your fears—somebody who will listen to you, talk to you, and try to help you deal with them realistically. Even if you can't pinpoint a specific fear, these techniques will greatly help you cope with general anxiety.

LEARN MORE ABOUT OSTEOARTHRITIS

Things that are unknown are often feared. And, unfortunately, there may still be a lot that you don't know about OA. However, the more people you speak to, the more questions you ask, and the more information you obtain, the fewer unknowns there will be. Knowledge is power! The more you know about OA, the course your disease may take, treatment options, and how to deal with pain, the easier it will be to eliminate many of your fears, or at least reduce them to a manageable level.

Let's Talk About Specifics

When you were first diagnosed, many fearful questions probably came to mind. "What will the future be like? What will become of me?" These are all typical questions of people who are diagnosed with any chronic medical problem, not just OA. As time went by, in all probability, some of these questions were answered and you started to adjust to having OA. But once these initial fears are reduced, others may arise. In other words, you may now focus on the fear of pain, concerns about reduced mobility, and worries of other possible symptoms, events, and experiences. All of these fears are normal and understandable, and should be expected. But however normal they may be, they can be harmful if you fail to cope with them effectively.

In the previous pages, we looked at some general coping strategies. But you're probably most interested in seeing how these and other strategies can help you better deal with the specific fears that you're struggling with right now as a result of your OA. Let's discuss some of these fears and see what methods of coping may help.

FEAR OF PAIN

Nobody likes pain. And because pain, unfortunately, is probably the most unpleasant problem associated with OA, you may be fearful of it. If you do feel pain, you'll wonder when you're going to feel some relief. You may fear each little twinge of pain, and interpret it as a sign that your condition is deteriorating or that additional problems exist or may develop.

What can you do about this fear? Try to accept the fact that you may experience some pain from time to time, but that medication and other interventions can reduce its intensity as well as its duration. Realize that each pain "cycle" will eventually stop, or at least ease up. The pain won't last forever. (For more suggestions on coping with pain, see Chapter 5.)

FEAR OF MEDICATION AND POSSIBLE SIDE EFFECTS

You may be nervous about the different medications that you have to take, even though you need them. You may be afraid of what they're doing to your body. Just keep reminding yourself what your OA would be like without medication! Your physician is aware of the possible side effects, but will still prescribe medication as long as the advantages of the medication outweigh the side effects.

FEAR OF "WHAT NEXT?"

What will happen next? Unfortunately, you can't be sure. Will there be an increase in the amount of pain? Will new joints be affected? Will you develop new side effects from your medication? Will you need joint replacement surgery? Fear of "what next?" includes being afraid of new problems, or the return of old ones.

Everyone *wonders* what's in store for the future. But because of OA, you may be *fearful* of the future, rather than merely curious. What can you do? Because you can't foresee what will happen in the future, take life one day at a time. Tell yourself that you'll handle any problems as they occur. Talk with others who have OA. Just keep doing what is necessary in order to take care of yourself.

FEAR OF DISABILITY

The thought of becoming disabled may be frightening. Because OA can be physically restricting, you may share this fear. But *disabled* is a bad term, since it suggests that you can't do anything. If you look around you and think more objectively, you will realize that having a physical disability won't make you any less of a human being. You will still have many, many capabilities. Numerous Olympic champions began their athletic careers to overcome physical disabilities. Beethoven wrote some of his greatest music after becoming totally deaf. Mickey Mantle played some of his best baseball despite arthritis-related pain. And "Broadway" Joe Namath had such problems with his knees that his football career was agonizing, although highly successful. So regardless of any restrictions from OA, be assured that you can overcome or at least compensate for a limitation in one area by developing or enjoying abilities in another.

How might a disability affect you? Maybe you'll be afraid of becoming increasingly dependent on others. But truthfully, it's your *thinking* that's making you afraid. Other than trying to take good care of yourself, what else can you really do? Take things as they come, but think more positively. Remember: You still have lots of room for self-fulfillment.

If you are already physically restricted, this can certainly be frightening, especially if you enjoy independence. You don't want to be a burden to those important people in your life. Can you do anything to prevent this? That depends on the nature of your restrictions. Find out everything you can about the possibility of rehabilitation. If there's any chance, take advantage of it. Even if there's no possibility of total rehabilitation, every little bit helps. Regardless, remember that you'd help someone you love if it were necessary. And the important people in your life care about you, don't they? So don't let yourself give up or you'll be doing yourself an enormous disservice. Fear of being totally unable to function crosses the minds of most people with OA at one time or another. But be assured that a great majority of the people with OA do *not* become totally incapacitated, even if they are not able to do as much as they used to do.

Your chances of needing a wheelchair are likewise small. It can happen, but only if your joints are very severely damaged—and this is most often a result of neglecting proper self-care. Advances in modern medicine continue to decrease the chances of becoming severely disabled as a result of OA. (This doesn't mean that on a trip to a place like Walt Disney World, you wouldn't welcome a wheelchair as a support device!).

FEAR OF FALLING

A very common fear for people with OA is that of falling down. There are two main reasons for this fear. First, you certainly don't want to hurt yourself. You may be afraid that if you fall, you'd really do a lot of damage. And, second, you may be afraid that, once you fall, you won't be able to get back up.

What can you do? Obviously, try to be as careful as possible. Try to avoid hasty movements. Use handrails whenever they are available. Reorganize your environment to reduce the chances of tripping over anything— for example, remove or secure throw rugs and keep traffic areas clear. Beyond this, however, remind yourself that you can do only so much. You don't want to fall. But if it happens, it happens, and you will deal with it!

FEAR OF THE REACTIONS OF OTHERS

Are you afraid that other people will react badly to you because of your osteoarthritis? Unfortunately, some people *can* be cold, unfeeling, and insensitive to your problems. But your true friends will accept you under any circumstances. Enjoy them.

Naturally, you should aim to live your life as normally as possible. Remain involved with family and friends. But be realistic. Remember that a change in a social relationship can occur for any reason, not just because of OA! And since you can't change the way some people feel, try not to be too concerned with their reactions. Instead, be more attentive to your own needs and feelings.

Of course, if you think that an important relationship is in jeopardy, you should try to figure out the reason and determine what you can do to improve things. And if you feel that people are shying away from you, try to discuss this with them. Find out what their concerns are. Maybe you'll be able to remedy the situation. Get counseling, if need be. But remember that you can do only so much. If your efforts don't work, at least you'll know that you did your best.

Finally, if you have been troubled by the reactions of others, you may find it helpful to get involved in a support group. You know that the people in these groups will not shy away from you or abandon you. Why? Because they're going through the same kinds of things that you are. And because of their own experiences, participants may even be able to give you some tips on dealing with family and friends. (For more information on dealing with others, see Chapters 20 to 26.)

FEAR OF OVERDOING OR UNDERDOING

You may not know how much you should be trying to accomplish. You may be afraid of doing too much, but feel guilty about doing too little. How can you conquer this fear? Get advice from experts. You'll need professional guidance to come up with the best mix of rest and exercise for you. And you'll need to know which, if any, activities may be too strenuous for you at certain times.

Of course, even your doctor may not have specific answers for you. You may be told that the answers will become apparent only through trial and error. After all, experience is the best teacher.

So what should you do? Pace yourself. Change your level of activity as needed, but try to change it gradually. One of the "advantages" of OA is that too much physical activity will signal you to slow down. Fortunately, rest can help painful joints feel better. Then tell yourself that, as with so many other fears, you're doing the best you can. Take pleasure in whatever you may accomplish.

FEAR OF EMPLOYMENT PROBLEMS

You may be concerned about the effect your condition will have on your job. You may want or need to work, but fear that symptoms will make it too difficult. Your employer may be understanding at first, but you'll probably worry about how long his or her tolerance will continue. And, of course, your need for money may be greater due to your medical problems. If you can't work, this pressure will be even greater.

What can you do? Talk to others who have been in the same situation, and see how they handled it. Speak to experts who can advise you on financial matters. Evaluate your vocational skills, and make sure you're equipped to do a job that you can physically handle. Remember, you'll work it out.

FEAR OF TRAVELING

You may be afraid to travel with OA. Why? You wouldn't know the doctors, what medical facilities were available, or whom you could contact if you experienced a problem. Obviously, if you travel by car, this may not be much of a problem. But you want to be sure you can walk as much as you'd like and that your environment is conducive to getting around.

What can you do? By planning in advance, you should be able to answer these concerns. Ask your physician if he or she knows of any doctors or facilities in the area where you're planning to go. You might want to contact them in advance. If your physician has no contacts, either try to get some names on your own (try the local medical society or your local chapter of the Arthritis Foundation) or plan your vacation at a place where adequate medical services are available. Plan on not overdoing. After all, visiting five landmarks in one day is a bit much!

FEAR OF NOT COPING

You may feel that you're barely handling your OA. You may believe that any new problem or symptom that comes along will be enough to push you over the edge. And fear of falling apart can easily lead to panic: an out-of-control feeling that can actually make this happen.

So get ahold of yourself. Pinpoint those particularly difficult things and get help in dealing with them. Don't wait, and don't project a false sense of bravado. If you feel yourself nearing the edge, get someone to help you steady yourself. Talk over your fears with someone. Once you have shared them, you may see things a little more clearly. You may be able to deal with problems with greater strength, knowing that you're not alone. And once you're back in control, your fear will disappear.

FEAR OF FEAR ITSELF

This section might be called "Fear of Anxiety," or "Fear of Panic Attacks," or any of a number of other things. What they all describe, though, is the response that many people have to bouts of anxiety and fear. Because these emotions are so uncomfortable, many people develop a fear of being afraid. This is known as a secondary anxiety reaction. It means that you're not afraid of a specific object, person, or situation as much as you're anxious about being anxious.

What to do? Start by using relaxation techniques. Then tell yourself that you will approach any situation or feeling as it occurs, rather than worrying about what might or might not happen. Reread the information in this chapter. And, if necessary, work with a supportive professional to help you better cope with this problem.

What Professional Treatments Are Available?

We've discussed a number of ways to deal with your anxieties and fears. The first step is to pinpoint what may be triggering them and see if you can change, or even eliminate, these triggers. (If you can't pinpoint them at the time you're anxious, at least try to do so once you've calmed down.) Then desensitize yourself to the source of your fears. You'll want to talk your feelings over with others to gain a fresh perspective. One very good way to increase your sense of control is to use relaxation techniques. Work on your thinking, to restructure any negative thoughts that may be contributing to, or exacerbating, the anxiety. And you'll want to learn more about your condition so that you can eliminate any fears of the unknown.

In some cases, using these techniques will bring about a sufficient degree of control. However, there may be times when you need additional help. Let's look at the types of professional treatments that are available.

MEDICATION

Medication is one means of treating intense fears or panic. The medications used are designed to block whatever is biochemically contributing to the onset or exacerbation of panic. Although certain drugs may be beneficial in dealing with panic attacks, they may not be appropriate for the less severe anxiety and fear most often associated with OA. If you feel that medication may be the answer for you, be sure to speak to your doctor. You will also want to make sure that any medications prescribed for anxiety or panic are compatible with your OA treatment. (For more information on medications, see Chapter 6.)

BEHAVIOR THERAPY

Because fear or panic may lead to additional anxieties and phobias, psychological techniques involving behavior therapy may be quite helpful.

For example, techniques such as systematic desensitization, discussed earlier in the chapter, can be very effective in reducing phobias. Behavior therapies are based on the principle that undesirable or inappropriate behaviors such as anxiety have been learned, and can therefore be unlearned and replaced with more appropriate, constructive ones. A qualified therapist should be able to help you better cope with your fears using this technique.

PSYCHOTHERAPY

Because intense fear or panic may throw you out of control, you may require professional intervention—especially if these attacks have been occurring often. In psychotherapy, a professional works with you to help you learn why your fears and anxieties exist, what may maintain them, and what techniques can help you defuse them. Psychologists, psychiatrists, and certified social workers are among the types of professionals that can practice psychotherapy. Don't feel that you are weak if you decide to consult a professional. After all, your goal is to feel better, right? So if you're having difficulty resolving some of these problems yourself, isn't it good to know that there are experts who can help you regain control?

A Fearless Summary

Although many different fears have been discussed in this chapter, we probably haven't covered all of the ones you could possibly experience. In addition, the coping suggestions offered certainly don't include all possible ways of dealing with fear. So what should you do?

Anticipate that you will fear certain things from time to time. Some fears will return, but plan on riding through them rather than succumbing to them. Not only is it okay to be scared, it's normal. Also remember that the most important thing is to overcome these fears so that they don't overwhelm you.

You're working on recognizing your fears, right? For some of them, you're modifying your behavior. For others, you're modifying your think-ing. Soon you will feel more in control. As this happens, you'll notice your fears begin to diminish. That doesn't mean that they'll all go away. But as you work on them, they will at least lessen in intensity, and you'll feel bet-ter knowing that you can handle whatever comes along.

CHAPTER SIXTEEN

Anger

Dolores, age 62, was fed up. She was tired of joint pain. She was tired of the medical visits. She was sick of hearing that there was nothing her doctor could do to eliminate her OA. From her doctor to her husband, practically everyone who went near her received an earful. What made her even more angry was that she wanted to slam her fist down on her kitchen table, but she knew it would just make her pain worse. Was Dolores angry? You bet your eardrums she was!

People with any chronic medical problem may be angry. It is certainly very common to feel anger when you have OA. But because anger results in a buildup of physical energy that needs to be released, it's important to learn how to cope with this emotion.

Just what is anger? When you have a desire or goal in mind and something interferes with efforts to reach it, this can be very frustrating. A feeling of tension and hostility may result, which is what we refer to as anger.

You may feel anger toward OA itself, toward your body, toward the medical profession, toward family and friends, even toward God or the universe. Virtually anybody or anything may be a target of your anger during your experience with OA. Sometimes it is even an outward manifestation of deeper emotional feelings that are more difficult to express, such as helplessness and frustration.

Are There Different Types of Anger?

In learning to deal with anger, it can be helpful to discuss three different ways in which anger can be experienced. This will enable you to more easily identify anger when it does occur.

The first type of anger is rage—the expression of violent, uncontrolled anger. If Dolores was feeling upset about her OA and a friend told her that her joints would still be healthy if she had drunk three glasses of milk each day, you can imagine how angry Dolores might become. Her anger might even lead her to say or do things that would certainly not enhance the prospects of a long-lasting, friendly relationship with this person. This is probably the most intense anger you can experience. It is an outward expression, since there is noticeable evidence of an explosion. Often, rage is a destructive release of intense physical energy that has built up over time.

The second type of anger is resentment. This feeling of anger is usually kept inside. What if Dolores listened to her friend's well-meaning comments, smiled, and said nothing, but was seething inside? This is resentment—a growing, smoldering feeling of anger, directed toward a person or object, but often kept bottled up. Resentment tends to sit uncomfortably within you and can do even more physiological and psychological damage than rage.

The third type of anger is indignation, a more appropriate, positive type of anger. Unlike rage, it is released in a controlled way. If Dolores had responded to her friend's comments by firmly stating that she appreciated the concern but would prefer no advice at this point, this would have been an expression of indignation.

Obviously, these three types of anger can occur in combination with each other and in many different ways. Understanding the different ways of experiencing anger can help you identify and cope with it when it does occur.

What Causes Anger?

There are, of course, lots of things that can make you angry. You may get angry if you keep breaking dishes because you can't hold them securely. You may get angry if you feel that the prescribed treatment isn't helping you. You may get angry if you have to wait to see your doctor. Or you may become angry if you feel that your family is not understanding enough.

Thoughtless comments from others can cause anger as well. "If you didn't play so much tennis, your joints would still be working!" This is not the kind of comment that would make you feel friendly. If you sense that someone is taking advantage of you, or if you feel forced to do something that you don't want to, anger may result. If you do not have the ability or confidence to say no when friends ask for a favor, this, too, can create feelings of anger—especially if you are feeling too fatigued to complete even your own tasks.

When thinking about the causes of anger, there may not be any specific reason you can point to. Or you might be able to list dozens of reasons. Being aware of this is important, because you must become aware of anger before you can deal with it. Unfortunately, resolving your anger won't make your OA go away. Nor should you say that you'd stop being angry only if your OA goes away. Neither attitude will help you.

In their anger over having OA, one of the most common questions that people ask is "Why me?" This question suggests that what happened shouldn't have happened—that it's unfair, or that someone or something is somehow to blame. Again, it's important to realize that in this case, anger is not helpful—that asking "Why me?" will not benefit you in any way. It's far better to ask yourself what you can do about it now that it has happened.

Before we finish looking at the causes of anger, it is important to realize that anger exists uniquely in the mind of each angry individual. Anger is a direct result of your thoughts, not of events. An event in and of itself does not make you angry. Rather, your anger is caused by your interpretation of the event—the way you think or feel about it. This is a very important point, and one that will be discussed in much more detail a little bit later.

How Does Anger Affect Your Body?

When you are angry, a number of physiological responses occur. Your breathing becomes more rapid, your blood pressure increases (you may feel as if your blood is "boiling"), and your heart may begin to pound. Your face may get hot and your muscles may tense. You may also feel stronger when angry. The more intense the anger, the greater is this feeling of power. In fact, you may be able to remember a time when you were so angry that you almost felt you had superhuman strength.

Anger is a form of energy. The more physical energy that builds up in the body due to anger, the more necessary it becomes to release it. This energy cannot be destroyed. So if it is not released in some constructive manner, it will eventually come out in another, less desirable way.

Imagine the energy from anger to be a stick of dynamite about to explode. If you get rid of it, it may cause some damage when it explodes, but it won't hurt you as much as it would if you swallowed it to keep others from getting hurt. Obviously, the ideal solution is to neither throw nor swallow the dynamite, but to defuse it. (More about defusing later in this chapter.)

Extreme anger usually passes quickly. If, however, the anger lasts for a long period of time, it can have physically damaging effects on the body. You've probably heard about some of the physical problems that can result from holding anger in, such as hypertension or headaches. Well, anger can also make your OA worse. How? Anger causes you to tense up, putting extra (and undesirable) pressure on your joints and muscles. It's just not good for your body. And remember, increased tension also leads to increased pain.

How Does Anger Affect Your Mind?

Anger is usually experienced as a very unpleasant feeling. However, it sometimes exists along with a more pleasurable feeling of power or strength. Frequently, the unpleasantness of anger is related to its consequences—knowing what you do when you are angry, and not being happy about it. Sometimes anger may become so extreme that you feel like exploding. You may feel that unless you are able to punch, kick, or hit something—to get rid of the anger in some way—you will lose control. Hopefully this angry energy can be released without causing damage to another person, property, or yourself. If, when you finally calm down, you find that you have done something destructive, you may become angry all over again. Or you may experience another negative emotion, such as guilt.

Is Anger Good or Bad?

Is anger ever good or constructive? "Avoid anger at all costs," many say, "because nothing good can come of it." But this is true only if you don't deal with anger properly. Anger can, indeed, be dangerous if it's kept inside or released in inappropriate ways.

Remember that stick of dynamite? What an explosive example! If anger is released in destructive ways, it can cause problems in relationships—to say the least! It can also aggravate your OA-related problems. Does this mean that anger can make your condition worse? Sure. What if you're so angry at somebody or something that you decide not to take proper care of yourself? For example, if you don't get enough rest, or you don't do the prescribed amount of exercise? What if you're so angry at somebody—perhaps your doctor or an overprotective friend—that you do more than you should? "I'll show them," you say. And then you go on to exhaust yourself. In this case, anger is obviously harmful, but only because you've turned it against yourself.

How can anger be constructive? First, it can give you an indication that something is wrong—something that needs attention. Second, it can motivate you to deal more actively with life's problems. Anger can give you a feeling of power or strength, of confidence or assertiveness. I'm not saying that you should slam your finger with a hammer or tell someone to punch you in order to make you angry enough to solve all of your problems. What I am saying is that anger can be positive and, if used correctly, can help you find solutions to real problems.

Some Different Reactions to Anger

Marie, a 52-year-old teacher, was having a hard time with her husband. He was trying to show concern for his wife by relieving her of some responsibilities around the house. But most days she felt well enough to continue doing her household chores, and wanted to be treated as normally as possible. She wanted to be the one to determine what she could and could not do. But Marie's husband couldn't see this, and Marie was running out of patience. Let's look at three ways in which this situation might be handled.

THE "JUST IGNORE IT" APPROACH

If you feel overwhelmed by the intensity of your anger, and fear that you may completely lose control, you may try to do whatever you can to avoid the experience. This might include pushing any angry thoughts out of your mind, no matter how important the issue.

So rather than focusing on household responsibilities, Marie could think about other activities and try not to show her resentment. Or she could try to appease her husband and agree with everything he said. This would at least be temporarily effective in helping Marie to cope. In the long run, however, you can see that this would not be the best way for Marie to deal with her anger.

THE "TAKE ACTION" APPROACH

It's possible to see anger as a necessary, though unpleasant, part of life. You know that there will be times when you'll be angry, whether you like it or not. But you can choose to deal with both your anger and the situation that's causing it as effectively as possible.

For example, Marie knows that she's not happy being angry, and might decide to speak to her husband so that he could better understand her emotional needs. In this case, even if Marie failed to persuade her husband to understand her need to assume most of her normal household responsibilities, she would at least have the satisfaction of knowing that she did something about her feelings.

THE "TAKE POWER" APPROACH

Maybe you enjoy the flow of energy and strength that comes from being angry. You may find that when you're angry, you are best able to assert yourself and get things done.

Marie might know that if smothered once too often, she would explode. She might love the feeling of power that this anger gives her. She might almost look forward to the chance to say, "Honey, if you treat me that way once more, I'll take this vacuum cleaner and . . . !"

If you enjoy this feeling, it is possible that you may even provoke situations to make yourself angry. Perhaps you've heard of professional basketball or tennis players who psych themselves up before a confrontation with an opponent. For them, getting angry is the best preparation for a successful performance!

Your own reaction to anger is unique. It may also change from time to time. There may be times when you accept anger and almost value it as a motivator. At other times you may attempt to push it away. Marie might enjoy expressing her anger. But if she didn't want to hurt her husband or upset the rest of the family, she might choose to have a calm discussion rather than shattering everyone's eardrums with an explosive confrontation.

Of course, the way in which you deal with your emotions now is probably similar to the way in which you've dealt with adversity in the past. If you have always dealt with problems in a generally positive, constructive manner, you will probably deal with new problems in the same way. On the other hand, if you have had difficulty dealing with stress in the past, you may also have problems dealing with it now. But remember that you can learn how to effectively cope with anger.

How Can You Cope with Anger?

You've now begun to realize that anger can be constructive. In order for anger to be helpful, there are some very important things to keep in mind. First, don't let yourself become overwhelmed by anger. Once that happens, it is much harder to do what you have to do. Second, don't be afraid of your anger. If you do fear it, you probably won't be able to release it properly. More than likely, it will come out in unhealthy ways, or you'll bottle it up inside. Third, be sure that the way you handle your anger is socially acceptable. Marie might get a kick out of knocking out her husband's teeth, but would the dentist (or the police) approve? Try to be flexible enough to recognize an appropriate way of releasing your anger.

Hopefully, the information you've read so far has been encouraging. But what else, specifically, can you do to cope with your own anger? Because anger is such a complex emotion, and because there are so many things that cause it, there are no simple answers. (Sorry about that!) Does this mean that there is nothing anybody can do about anger? No. You can do a lot to reduce your feelings of anger and to handle them more efficiently, comfortably, and safely.

First, of course, you must be able to admit that you're angry, and you must figure out *why*. Once you've pinpointed the source of your anger, you may be able to defuse it or, if that's not possible, to find an acceptable outlet. Let's take a look at each of these ways of coping with anger.

RECOGNIZE YOUR ANGER

There are two steps involved in recognizing anger: admitting it exists and identifying the source. Let's look at these in greater detail.

Step One: Admit That You're Angry

The first step in dealing with anger is to recognize that you're angry. As simple as this may sound, many people cannot take this first step. They may try to deny it, or they may rationalize their feelings or behavior using other explanations.

Do you feel that being angry is a sign of weakness? If so, you may not admit that you're angry—perhaps not even to yourself. You may feel that there is no appropriate reason to be angry, and that it is a childish reaction. But, as with anything else, in order to change something, you have to first recognize that it exists.

How can you tell if you're angry? If you feel very tense (jumping at the sound of the telephone), or find yourself reacting with impulsiveness (slamming down the phone when you get a wrong number and storming out of the house), or become hostile (cursing at your neighbor for leaving a speck of garbage on your lawn), chances are that you're angry. Don't be afraid to recognize it—that this is the first step in dealing with it.

Step Two: Identify the Source of Your Anger

The second step in dealing with anger is trying to identify its source. Where did the anger come from? What is contributing to it? What events have led to these feelings of anger?

For one thing, as we mentioned earlier in the chapter, you could certainly be angry because you have OA. You may be angry with yourself for neglecting your condition. You might be angry at your physician, whether justifiably or not. You may be angry because you feel out of control. In some cases, the events leading to an angry reaction may be quite obvious. In other cases, however, it may be hard to pinpoint the cause. Keep probing—you will eventually find the source of the problem.

So it's necessary to explain to yourself *why* you're angry. Why is this step important? Because you want to decide whether or not the anger you're feeling is realistic. If necessary, write down what you think is making you feel this way. Be honest when writing down your thoughts, regardless of how violent or profane they may be. Rich, colorful language can be helpful in releasing your feelings, and will ultimately allow you to control your anger. Try to examine your thoughts objectively, the way someone else might look at them. If you recognize that your reasons are understandable, this alone may help you deal with your feelings. Your next step will be to decide how you can best handle them.

Now, depending on the situation, you can either defuse your anger or find an appropriate outlet for it. Read on to see how each of these techniques can work for you.

DEFUSE YOUR ANGER

In the past, many people believed—incorrectly—that there were only two possible ways to deal with anger: to either keep it inside or let it out. But what about a third possibility? Remember when we talked about defusing that stick of dynamite? Your anger is a result of the way you think. In your mind, you are interpreting events in a way that makes you angry. So if you can change the way you interpret things and reorganize your thinking patterns, you can actually stop creating the anger that you feel.

Is this really possible? Well, if something happened that made you angry, would everybody in the world be angry because of it? No. Only you would feel this way. Others might not be angry because their interpretation of the event would be different. Let's look at some of the ways that you can defuse your anger *before* it becomes a problem.

Watch Mental Movies

When you become angry, you frequently have all kinds of pictures in your head—images of what's making you angry and of how you'd like to deal with your feelings. These "mental movies" help you defuse your anger.

For example, imagine that you're in tremendous pain and very tired. Your friend calls to tell you that her car has broken down. Could you please pick up her dry cleaning? When you tell her that your joints are too sore to pick up lint, much less dry cleaning, she says something about how she can never depend on you for anything. This is a friend? You become irate. At that moment, ask your friend to hold on, close your eyes, and imagine all the abusive things you'd like to say to her. Then imagine the shocked expression on her face. By using this mental imagery, you'll probably be able to complete the phone call without destroying a friendship. You may even smile or laugh as you think about the scenes playing through your mind. (See Chapter 5.)

Ruth was quite annoyed with her husband, Messy Max. Whenever she asked for his help around the house, he was grouchy and uncooperative. Just before Ruth was about to give him a haircut with a meat cleaver, she remembered the mental movie technique. She imagined herself strangling him—his eyeballs popping out and gurgling sounds coming from his throat. This helped to rid Ruth of the intense, angry feelings that were making her crazy, and allowed her to deal with Max more constructively. (No, she's not in jail.)

Ruth was lucky in that she was eventually able to enlist her husband's help. She even made a deal with him—she would let him watch football games without the kids interfering as long as he agreed to help her. But even if Ruth realized that she would not be able to change her husband's behavior, that very realization would have been constructive. How? It would have allowed Ruth to move on and seek solutions that didn't require her husband's help. (For more information on dealing with others, see Chapters 20 through 26.)

Picture a Big Red Stop Sign

Another technique that can help you to control your anger is "thought stopping." Remember: It is the thoughts in your mind that are making you angry—the thoughts you have when you interpret an event. So when you find that angry thoughts have come into your head, picture a big red stop sign. Seeing that picture in your mind will serve as a momentary distraction. Then concentrate on something you enjoy. This can be a peaceful, relaxing scene; a type of food you like; or a favorite movie or television program. Whatever you choose, you will divert your thinking and give your anger a chance to dissipate. You could also participate in a pleasant distracting activity—reading a book, taking a walk, taking a relaxing bath, or calling a friend, for instance. Any of these activities should help defuse your anger.

Change Your Requirements

At times, you may have specific requirements—particular ways that you want certain things to occur. When these needs are not met, you may feel angry. Modifying your demands can help you cope with your anger.

Let's say that you're not feeling well and decide to call your doctor. The answering service tells you that she is not in the office and that you should get a return call within half an hour. After forty-five minutes, the doctor has not yet returned your call, and you are fuming. Why? Because your requirement of having your call returned within thirty minutes was not met.

What can you do? Revise your expectations. Tell yourself that you would have liked a call within thirty minutes, but that your doctor may be in surgery, with another patient, in transit, or simply unable to get to a phone. You'll be satisfied if you get a call at her earliest convenience. By modifying your requirement, you'll feel less angry.

Another way to benefit from this technique is to write down your expectations. Then try to revise them with new, more flexible ones. This may help you see your requirements in a more objective light.

Put Yourself in the Other Person's Shoes

One of the best ways of dealing with anger toward another person is to try to understand exactly what he or she is feeling, wants, or is saying. This will help you accept the behavior and deal with it more constructively. This technique can also help you understand how that other person will feel if he or she is the target of your abusive release of anger.

Jerry got angry when his wife insisted that they go out for dinner when he got home from work. He was in pain, and the last thing on his mind was food. It had been hard enough for him to get through the day. Now all he wanted to do was stay home and relax. Jerry knew that he had to find a better way to handle his anger. So rather than exploding, he imagined what his wife was feeling—how disappointed she was because, after all, she loved trying new restaurants and going out with him. Jerry's new under-

standing let him defuse his anger and explain why he couldn't always ac-
company her, even though he wished he felt like going.

LET YOUR ANGER OUT

We have now looked at a number of ways to control your thinking and improve your ability to interpret events to keep your anger from growing. But
these techniques may not always be successful. What if there are times
when you remain angry? How can you deal with anger in a constructive
way when you just can't defuse it? Fortunately, there are two possibilities.
Let's see what these are.

Talk, Don't Bite

Obviously, it is much more desirable to discuss an issue constructively
than to have an angry exchange of heated words, accomplishing nothing.
In most cases, anger arises when you have a conflict or problem with another person. For this reason, it can be very helpful to learn ways to nego-
tiate a solution. Remember that a heated argument—fighting fire with
fire—is not the answer. Instead, you want to put out the fire by reducing
the heatedness of the argument.

How can you do this? Try complimenting the person, or looking for
positive things that person is saying. Yes, you can do this even though
you're angry. This will work in two ways. First, it will probably surprise the
person. How will this help? Well, part of what fuels the fire of anger is your
anticipation of the other person's anger. So by catching that person off
guard, and thereby preventing an angry reaction, you will reduce the
flames. Second, by focusing on words or thoughts that are more constructive, you will calm yourself rather than letting your anger grow. And once
you're calm, you'll be able to quietly state your feelings.

Let's take our earlier example in which you became upset by your
friend's request to pick up her dry cleaning. Instead of blowing up and
telling her how inconsiderate she is, say that she was right to call you—
that you're glad she thought of you. But then tell her that, as much as you
would like to do this favor for her, you are not physically able to do it. Re-

gardless of what she says, keep looking for a positive way to respond, and continue to calmly indicate that you don't feel well. Eventually, you'll get your point across. Although she may not be too happy about it—she may even become angry—you will have resolved a problem constructively.

Write Out Your Anger

There are times when something or someone makes you so angry that you feel as if you're going to explode. You recognize the need to release these feelings because they're damaging to you, but you don't have the confidence to speak up. This would be a great time to write an angry letter. Writing can be a constructive way of diffusing this intense anger without damaging any relationships in the process. For example, you could write to your doctor, your partner, your neighbor, the medical profession, the "powers above," even your OA—virtually anyone, real or not, with whom you feel angry. But remember that for this technique to work best, *don't* let anyone see your letter! After you finish pouring your venom onto paper, destroy it. You'll be destroying some of your anger at the same time!

Find a Physical Release for Your Anger

In general, one of the best outlets for releasing angry energy is physical activity. But what if this is not an option, because of OA, your age, or any other reason? Fortunately, there are solutions.

Some people find that they can release the physical energy from anger by *watching* things! For example, watching a sporting event may help you to release anger by getting you mentally involved in the activities you're viewing. Or you might try watching an emotionally draining movie. You may become so totally absorbed that your built-up energy is released through worry, fear, or excitement. A book that allows you to identify with the characters can be beneficial as well—especially if the characters themselves release anger.

Believe it or not, another common and very effective outlet for anger is crying. We're sure you've heard about the therapeutic effects of a good cry. Although this technique is not for everyone, if your anger has built up to the point of uncontrollable crying, this can be a great way to let it out. (Of course, you may scare the daylights out of your family. But just tell them you read about it here!)

Some people like to count to ten when angry. This may distract you from what is causing you to feel this way and give you a chance to calm down and think about it more constructively. Try counting out loud, and expressing your feelings through facial expressions and tone of voice. Count to a thousand, if necessary!

An Anger-Free Summary

It is important to remember that events alone do not make you angry. Rather, how you think and interpret these events is what leads to anger. And since it is your thinking that makes you angry, you have contributed to feeling this way. So you must be responsible and begin helping yourself cope with anger—or, at least, reducing it to a more manageable level.

The best way to handle anger is to remain in control so that it doesn't build up—to restructure your thinking so that your emotions don't get out of hand. But if anger does build, remember that when channeled and used constructively, it can be beneficial. And when this isn't possible, you can defuse or release your anger in a harmless way.

CHAPTER SEVENTEEN

Guilt

Have you ever felt guilty? Many people who have OA say that they have. In fact, family members may feel guilt as well.

Certainly, guilt is a very unpleasant feeling. Take the case of Rosie. She was very unhappy because she couldn't knit sweaters for her grandchildren anymore. She felt she wasn't being the kind of grandmother she wanted to be. Why not? Well, because she just couldn't participate in enough activities with her grandchildren. So having OA made her feel guilty that she was being a bad grandmother. Was it hard for her to cope with this guilt? You bet! But Rosie didn't have to be a victim of this emotion. Let's first take a look at what leads to guilty feelings, and then explore some techniques you can use to help overcome them. After all, you want to do everything possible to make yourself feel better, and it's hard to feel good when you're feeling guilty.

What Are the Components of Guilt?

Feelings of guilt usually have two components. The first of these is the sense of *wrongdoing*—the feeling that you have either done something wrong or haven't done something that you should have done. The second component is the feeling of *badness* that results from this self-blame. It's this second component that's the true culprit. When you feel bad about doing something wrong, this is normal and understandable. But when you start telling yourself that you are a bad person, guilt follows.

What Causes Guilt?

There are a lot of things related to your OA that might make you feel guilty, even though there's probably no validity to any of them. For example, maybe you're concerned that something you did caused your OA. You may, for instance, feel guilty because you didn't take care of yourself properly, perhaps waiting too long before going to the rheumatologist. You could feel that if it weren't for certain actions—or lack of actions—on your part, you would not be in this situation. Or you may feel guilty simply because you are not able to find any rational reason for the disease. Therefore, you blame yourself.

You may also feel guilty if you think that you're complicating matters for your family as a result of your OA. You may worry that you're not going to be able to do all that is expected of you. You may feel guilty about letting yourself down or about disappointing others, whether they be family, friends, or colleagues. Guilt may also result because you are jealous of others who do not have OA, and then feel bad about that.

Perhaps others have told you that your feelings have no rational basis, that you're not at fault. Unfortunately, this may not eliminate guilt. Why? Because your feelings may have nothing to do with what others say or think. Remember: Your guilt comes from your own beliefs that you are a bad person.

Obviously, guilt can be a destructive emotion. It can drain you physically and emotionally, and can undermine your efforts to cope successfully with OA. Fortunately, there's plenty you can do to improve your outlook. In the remainder of this chapter, we'll look at the various techniques you can use to cope with this emotion.

How Can You Cope with Guilt?

Regardless of the cause of your guilt—and whether or not it is a new or long-standing problem for you—there are a number of strategies that can help you reduce or eliminate this unpleasant and harmful emotion. Let's take a look at some of the best ways.

FIND THE SOURCE OF YOUR GUILT

In order to successfully cope with guilt, you must first focus on what led to the guilty feelings in the first place. Sometimes just by pinpointing the source of this emotion, you can greatly reduce or even eliminate it.

For example, ask yourself if you have actually done something wrong. If you really believe that this is true, then ask yourself if your behavior was really so terrible. In Rosie's case, she felt guilty because her OA restricted her activities. Does that make sense? Did she make it happen? Of course not. So identify the cause of your guilty feelings and examine the wrong-doing you think you committed. You will probably find either that you are not responsible for the wrong action, or that it was really not terrible enough to justify feeling so guilty.

Sometimes people feel guilty about thoughts or desires, rather than specific actions or behaviors. Recognize the difference between feeling guilty over a thought and feeling guilty over an action. Then, once you've identified the thought that's making you feel like a bad person, change it. Learn to talk to yourself in a positive way. Look at thoughts objectively and constructively in order to reduce your guilt.

But what if you feel guilty and simply can't remember what you were thinking or doing that made you feel this way? How can you use all the great thought-changing ideas we're going to talk about if you can't identify the ones you want to change? Good question! In order to pinpoint these "target" thoughts or behaviors, you might want to keep a brief written log of feelings or activities that may be causing your guilt. Once you have recorded them, you can begin to determine the root of the problem and then think about what changes might improve the situation.

TALK IT OVER

It's very important to discuss your feelings about having OA with others who may be affected by it. Share your concerns, and try to figure out solutions to any problems that exist.

Jane, a 58-year-old woman who had been married for over thirty years, enjoyed going square dancing with her husband twice each week. (No squares, these two!) In addition, she and her husband would participate in other social activities with friends at least one or two other evenings each week. Now, because of the pain she was experiencing from OA, she had to restrict her activities. She just couldn't go out as frequently. She couldn't even do-si-do her partner! Sometimes, she wouldn't want to go out even once during an entire week. Not only did she feel unhappy about her condition, but she felt extremely guilty about holding her husband back. She felt that he couldn't have a good time because of her.

Fortunately, Jane had the good sense to sit down with her husband and discuss the situation. Together they decided that until Jane regained some of her strength, she would rest at home while her husband would get involved in other physical activities with friends. To end their discussion on a positive note, together they decided that when she felt better they would go to Atlantic City. Jane felt better knowing that her limitations would not prevent her husband from enjoying activities. And Jane also had something to look forward to—a fun trip with her husband.

TURN YOUR THOUGHTS AROUND

Is there anything you can do about the negative thoughts that lead to guilt—those thoughts that make you feel that you're a bad person? One helpful thing to do is try to restructure your thinking to make it more positive and guilt-free. Recognize that if you haven't done anything to lead to guilt, you should identify those thoughts that are making you feel like a bad person. Change them. If you can learn to talk to yourself in a positive way, looking at your thoughts objectively and constructively, guilt can be reduced.

For example, let's say that you feel guilty because you believe that you're not being a good partner. Ask yourself if you've ever done anything that a good partner might do. Just about every person in a relationship can name many things. This type of thinking will begin to eliminate your "bad partner blues." The idea is to turn your mind's negative thoughts into reasonable, positive ones. This way, the feeling of guilt will not take a stranglehold.

REEVALUATE YOUR GOALS

Do you see a difference between the way you are doing something and the way you think you *should* be doing it? If so, you are probably feeling guilty! How can you work this out? Can you work harder or do more? If you can, and it's appropriate for you to do so, then you've solved your problem. If not, try examining your day-to-day goals for working and living. Ask yourself if these goals are practical, considering what you can and cannot do because of your OA.

When evaluating your goals, you may find that among the most common causes of guilt are thoughts containing the word *should. Should* is a dirty word! For example, you may think that you *should* be able to work harder and earn more money. Other *should* thoughts might include, "I should have been able to finish cleaning that room today," and, "I really should be helping my wife around the house today." These *should* thoughts imply that you must be just about perfect and right on top of everything. Naturally, you will become upset whenever you fall short of your *should.* But are you to blame when *should* thoughts establish goals that are unrealistic—goals that you may not be able to fulfill? Obviously, the answer is no!

Now that we've explained what you shouldn't do, what exactly should you do? In order to feel better and reduce guilt, reword your thoughts to eliminate the word *should.* Use less demanding ones. Say, "It would be nice if I could finish that task today, but I can't," rather than, "I should finish that task today." If you have trouble changing the wording of your *should* thoughts, try asking yourself, "Why should I . . . ?" or "Who says I should . . . ?" or "Where is it written that I should . . . ?" This may help you decide whether you are setting up impossible requirements for yourself and help you reduce your guilt feelings.

Let's say, for example, that you are thinking of having a party because all of your friends have invited you to get-togethers. Ask yourself why you should feel obligated to reciprocate. Is it because the "Party Rulebook" tells you that if you don't have a party, your friendship license will be revoked? Is it because if you don't have a party, your friends—some friends!—won't invite you to their homes anymore? As you think of some realistic answers to these questions, it will be easier to realize that you don't have to entertain. Although it would be nice, it would be more sensible to wait until you're feeling better.

Another way to eliminate guilt feelings over *should* thoughts is to take more pride in what you *can* do, rather than focusing on things you feel you should do but can't. Although most people hate hearing that "things could be worse," in the case of OA, this may be quite true. However, if you concentrate on what you are able to do, rather than on the negative, your feelings of guilt will diminish and you'll feel a lot better. Changing your thinking will also help you reduce the perceived gap between what is real and what you feel "should" be—which is what led to your guilty feelings in the first place.

ESCAPE FROM ESCAPE BEHAVIOR

So far, we have been discussing what leads to guilt, how you may feel, and how you can try to adjust your thoughts and behaviors to feel better. But what happens if you have not yet been successful in eliminating guilt? Sometimes, people who fail to cope with their guilt act in negative ways to hide from their feelings. They may also indulge in "escape" behaviors, such as drinking or excessive sleeping. This behavior does not confront problems head-on, but instead attempts to push them away.

Joe, a sixty-seven-year-old bookkeeper, felt guilty because he had stopped making plans with his friends. He did this because he could no longer hold playing cards in his hands, and felt that his friends would no longer be interested in getting together with him. As a result, he did begin to lose friends, and his guilt became more and more difficult to bear. He began drinking each day, in an attempt to escape and forget his misery. This behavior did not help the situation. In fact, it was downright dangerous. Not only did it compound the problem, but there was the added danger of mixing alcohol and medication. Now Joe had something else to feel guilty about: his escape behavior. This could increase his feeling of badness, leading to even more guilt and creating a vicious circle.

As you may have already guessed, the first step toward improvement is to look past the escape behavior and identify what is causing the guilt. Then consider what can be done to rectify the problem. At the same time, try to eliminate the escape behavior, recognizing that this activity is not improving your situation in any way. If, for example, Joe's physical condition kept him from holding playing cards, aren't there devices that could do this for him? Or does he really believe that his friends would want to see him only if he were a cardplayer? That would be ridiculous.

If you have difficulty doing this by yourself—or, for that matter, in identifying the root of the problem—by all means consider working with a supportive professional. You're worth it! It is possible, of course, that there is no clear-cut way to eliminate the situation or feelings that have led to your guilt. But don't give up. Instead, look for partial answers. This may not be as desirable as finding complete solutions, but it can still help reduce your guilt and make you feel better about yourself.

A Guiltless Summary

Guilt is a very destructive emotion—one that can interfere with your success in coping with OA by lowering your self-image and exhausting your emotional resources. By becoming aware of how guilt develops, pinpointing the source of your guilt, and changing your thinking to be more positive and realistic, you should be able to decrease or eliminate this feeling, and, instead, use your energy to successfully cope with your OA.

CHAPTER EIGHTEEN

Stress

Stress! Every time you turn around, you read or hear about stress. What exactly is it? Stress is a response that occurs in your body. It is a form of energy—a normal reaction to the demands of everyday life. It helps you mobilize your strength to deal with different events and circumstances.

Many things occur each day that require you to adapt. These are known as *stressors*. The changes that take place in your body when something (the stressor) provokes you are known as the *stress response*.

We all know that stress can play a role in causing or exacerbating virtually any medical problem. And OA is no exception. In fact, any experience with OA both causes and can be affected by stress.

What Are the Symptoms of Stress?

Your body will tell you when the stress you're experiencing is excessive. What might you feel? Physical signs include sweaty palms, heart palpitations, tightness of the throat, fatigue, nausea, diarrhea, or headaches—among other things. Emotionally, depression, anxiety, anger, frustration, or simply a vague uneasiness are just a few possible reactions. Of course, if OA causes any of these same symptoms, it might be hard to separate the two. So it is important is to tune into both your body and your mind to know when you can benefit from stress-reduction techniques.

Who Feels Stress?

Everyone experiences stress. Nobody escapes it. But since stress can be positive or negative, learning how to respond positively will lead to more stable emotional and physical states. If you have a hard time responding to stress, this won't be easy. Some people are more vulnerable to negative stress responses than others. Are you?

How Does Stress Affect You?

The effects of stress—much like the effects of depression, discussed in Chapter 14—are not isolated problems. Instead, they are part of a complex response that can involve both your body and your emotions. Let's examine this in more detail.

HOW STRESS AFFECTS YOUR BODY

Stress is a natural survival response. It occurs within the body whenever you feel threatened by thoughts or external pressures.

Stress can manifest itself in many ways. When you are in a stressful situation, your circulatory system works faster and blood is pushed rapidly toward different parts of the body—particularly to the protective organs and systems raising your blood pressure. Because the blood supply has been diverted to other organs, digestion is usually slowed. Stress also constricts the blood vessels, increases heart rate, and produces other physiological manifestations—all instantaneously!

What else can occur? Trembling and perspiring are very common reactions. Your face may flush. You may feel a surge of adrenaline flowing through your body. Your mouth may become dry and you may feel nauseated. Your breathing may become more rapid and shallow. Your heart may begin to pound. Your muscles may become tight, leading to headaches or cramps. Sounds wonderful, doesn't it?

So when you experience stress, your body prepares itself physiologically to counter any threat to its survival. Why? Perhaps you've heard of the *fight-or-flight response.* When an animal feels threatened, it prepares to either fight or run away. You will never see an animal standing there, scratching its head, and thinking about how to best handle the situation. Even though we have the ability to think and reason, we also experience the fight-or-flight response, which causes the secretion of many different hormones, and tenses the muscles in preparation for battle. If the response does involve physical action—fight or flight—the hormones are utilized as they are supposed to be, the muscles are exercised, and energy is released appropriately. However, if there is no physical exertion—if you *think* instead of taking action—the energy that was mobilized may not be released in the most appropriate way. This may explain why, after a period of stress during which you take no action, you feel exhausted just the same.

When does stress lead to physical problems? When you can't respond in a way that eliminates it, the stress continues unabated—and so do its symptoms. If you are not able to relieve the stress, you end up causing even more stress, creating a vicious cycle. And this can take its toll on your body. If stress is not controlled, it can make your OA even worse.

HOW STRESS AFFECTS YOUR MIND

Your emotional response to stress may not be as obvious as your physical response. You may start worrying, and fear the next "event." Your attention span is then reduced, and you are less able to concentrate on the task at hand. You may have trouble learning anything new and even be afraid to do things. You may withdraw or feel nervous. You may begin to lose confidence in yourself.

As you become nervous and upset, you are likely to notice some unpleasant physical responses you're experiencing, and this may make you feel even more stressed. For example, if you experience shallow, rapid breathing or heart palpitations, your awareness of these reactions may lead to feelings of panic. Most people respond to stress both physically and emotionally, although it is possible to respond in only one way. Do you have your own typical reaction? Maybe you become too jittery and unfocused to concentrate on your job. Perhaps you feel physically ill, with extreme intestinal discomfort, diarrhea, or a throbbing headache. Regardless of what you experience, it's important to learn strategies that will help you cope.

Three Reactions to Stress

We've just seen how your body and mind respond to stress. But we also want to look at a third type of response—the way you choose to deal with stress.

When a stressful stimulus occurs, you will most likely react in one of three ways. You might not respond at all and either "go with the flow" or become unable to function. You might respond immediately and impulsively, without giving thought to whether a better response might be possible. Or you might respond to stressors in a well-planned, organized, and effective manner. If so, you may not even need this chapter! But please read on!

Is Stress Good or Bad?

By now, you've probably figured out that stress can be either good or bad. If it gives you extra energy to do the things that you must do, then it is good. In fact, a certain amount of stress is normal and necessary. Stress helps you "get your act together," and prepares you to handle your life in the best possible way. But if left unchecked, stress can be highly destructive, draining all of your energy and possibly worsening your OA symptoms or any emotional problems. So while stress can be helpful, this chapter concerns itself with harmful stress—the kind that can hurt you if it goes uncontrolled.

What Causes Stress?

A number of things can act as stressors. Work-related problems, marital disputes, the death of a loved one, even some positive events such as a promotion at work or the arrival of a new baby—all can cause stress. But in this book, I am most concerned with the effects of OA on your life. Having osteoarthritis can cause stress in a number of different ways. For example, pain alone can cause stress. Concerns about whether your OA will get worse can cause stress. Worries about joint replacement surgery can be stressful. Problems with medication are also stressors. Worries about not being able to fulfill family or career responsibilities can cause stress. Side effects of medication, anticipation of surgery, fear of complications, adjustments to lifestyle changes, and financial and family pressures may also provoke a stress response.

Do events by themselves cause stress? And will the events that cause stress in one person necessarily cause it in another—and to the same degree? As you may have guessed, the answer is no. Why? Because, as with fear and anger, every person has a unique way of responding. Your reactions depend on a number of things. Your upbringing, your self-esteem, your beliefs about yourself and the world, the way in which you guide yourself in your thoughts and actions—all of these things help determine your response. How in control of your life you feel also plays an important role in this response. And your physical and emotional health—as well as your response to others—are also factors.

To sum it up, everyone's way of dealing with stress is unique and individual, and depends on a complex combination of thoughts and behaviors. To keep things simple, though, we can view the stress response as dependent on the chemistry between two factors. The first factor is the stressor, or the outside pressure. In other words, what is going on around you that is creating a problem? The second factor is your interpretation of the event. The interaction of the stressor and your internal interpretation together determine your response to stress. (Sound familiar? Yes, it's the same formula that can be applied to anger, depression, and any other emotion.) So the equation for the stress response can be depicted as follows:

Stressor + Interpretation = Stress Response

This equation has important implications for coping with stress. Why? Because it indicates that stress is not solely the result of your environment, OA, or any other factor around you. The way you interpret this stressor is of equal importance. Of course, some stressors would produce a negative response in anybody. What would happen, for example, if somebody pointed a knife at your throat? Calm acceptance, or a stress response? Get the point? In many situations, though, you do have the ability to control your reaction.

As you learn to cope with stress, it's important to remember that your mind responds to any threats as though they are real and happening right now. Any thoughts or images in your mind that produce a stress response are perceived as existing in the present, because the brain and the nervous system do not recognize the difference between past, present, and future. So it's easy to see that you contribute to your body's stress response with your own thoughts and images. This makes it even more important to feed your mind with the best, most beneficial, and most constructive information available.

How Can You Cope with Stress?

Because stress can affect the body and mind in so many ways, learning how to manage it is a very important part of any program for coping with OA. Not only can stress exacerbate the unpleasant and often debilitating symptoms of OA, but OA can cause enormous amounts of stress on physical, social, and psychological levels. The good news is that, regardless of how you have handled stress in the past, you can learn effective strategies that will help you effectively deal with it now. These strategies will make you feel more in control, lessening the feelings of anxiety and increasing your emotional well-being. And because of the mind-body connection, these strategies will also help your body better cope with OA.

But before we look at how you should cope with stress, let's look at what you *shouldn't* do. Smoking, alcohol abuse, the use of inappropriate drugs, and overeating are all common behaviors many individuals use, but they are poor coping strategies. True, these activities will distract you and perhaps delay the effects of the stress, but they can also hurt you and prevent you from coping with stress in a constructive way.

So what should you do? Try to learn new, more appropriate ways of dealing with stress. Relaxation techniques and regular exercise are important components of a stress management program. Thinking more appropriate and positive thoughts is also helpful. But be realistic and remember that while stress can be managed and controlled, it cannot be eliminated. Your focus, then, should be on using some of the following management techniques to help yourself deal better with both the physical and the emotional effects of stress.

USE RELAXATION TECHNIQUES

Because relaxation is incompatible with stress, the best way to start controlling stress is to use relaxation techniques. In fact, relaxation techniques alone—used without any other coping strategies—may allow you to successfully cope with both the physical and the emotional effects of stress.

Relaxation benefits you in many ways. First, it can give your body a chance to rest and recuperate. And a stronger body can help you deal better with the ravages of stress—and life!—and enable you to derive increased benefits from any medication you may be taking. Relaxation will also help you sleep better. Relaxation is also pleasurable, and will increase your feeling of emotional well-being. And it can give you a powerful sense of reestablishing control over your life, despite the presence of a chronic medical problem.

There are many different types of clinical relaxation techniques, including meditation, autogenics, and deep breathing. Hypnosis and biofeedback can also be used to induce relaxation, although they have other uses as well. (A full discussion of these and other relaxation techniques appears in Chapter 5.)

One relaxation technique that is often successful in combating stress is imagery—a technique that can also be used to cope with pain and other problems. Imagery is the process of formulating mental pictures or scenes in order to harness your body's energy and improve your physical or emotional well-being. In this case, of course, you will want to conjure up images that are relaxing and stress-free. Imagine not only the sights but also the smells, the tactile sensations (touch), and the sounds. The more vivid your image, the more helpful it will be. Feel comfortable with whatever degree of clarity your image takes on. The degree of relaxation you'll experience is up to you, and the degree to which you practice. You are in control. (More information about imagery in Chapter 5.)

PINPOINT THE SOURCE OF YOUR STRESS

Now that you're more relaxed, you're ready to objectively identify your stressors. What, specifically, is causing you to feel stress? Maybe you're having a hard time dealing with the never-ending pain of OA. Maybe you're concerned about medication. Perhaps you are concerned about the possibility of surgery. Of course, there are many more possibilities.

What if you're not sure what's causing your stress? How can you figure out what it is? Try keeping a log of your daily pressures. This will allow you to more easily recognize the people, places, and things that have the potential to create stress in your life. But what if you can't pinpoint which of your many activities are the real culprits? As you keep your log, you might want to use a numerical rating scale, such as the subjective units of disturbance (SUD) scale. How does it work? Ratings on this scale range from 0 to 100, depending on the amount of stress you're experiencing. Use 100 to represent the most extreme and disturbing stress, and 0 to represent no stress—total and complete relaxation. Then rate your activities, experiences, and thoughts. The ones with the higher SUD numbers are the ones causing you the most tension. (For example, loud music blasting from your neighbor's radio might be rated a whopping 85!)

IDENTIFY YOUR STRESS REACTIONS

Once you have begun identifying your stressors, you'll want to become completely aware of your responses to them. Are they more physiological or psychological? What parts of your body seem to be the most vulnerable? What specific reactions does your body have? Does your attention span suffer? Do you get heart palpitations? Do you start losing confidence, or feel as if you're "slipping"? As you become more aware of these things, you will develop a complete picture of your own unique stress response. This picture will help you choose the coping strategies that will be most useful in dealing with the events that trigger your stress.

ELIMINATE STRESSORS WHEN POSSIBLE

What's the next step? Once you recognize which stressors are causing the most trouble, try to determine whether or not you can eliminate them. Removing the source of the stress is an obvious and logical way to manage it. For instance, if the task of managing your household expenses is increasing your anxiety, you might have your spouse or another family member take over this chore. Obviously, different types of stressors would have to be removed in other ways.

CHANGE YOUR VIEW OF THE STRESSOR

What happens if you can't eliminate the source of your stress? You will then have to work on your interpretation of the stressors. You might want to use some of the suggestions discussed in Chapters 15 and 18. Or you might want to try systematic desensitization, discussed in Chapter 15.

Another technique that might help you cope better is *stress inoculation.* How can you be inoculated against stress? Well, you're certainly familiar with the use of inoculations to protect children from such diseases as measles. Exposing a child to the virus or other agent that causes a disorder prompts the child's body to develop an immunity to the disorder. Similarly, stress inoculation uses mental rehearsal procedures to help you confront and, gradually, tolerate stressful situations. As we saw earlier, because the mind responds to thoughts and mental images as if they were real and happening right now, thinking about something can be just as stressful as experiencing it. So by learning to cope with a situation in your mind, you can learn to deal with it in real life before it even happens.

Start your stress inoculation process by using whatever relaxation techniques you have found most helpful. Once you have achieved a comfortable level of relaxation, start imagining one of the stressors you've previously identified. As you imagine the stressful scene, recognize any physiological sensations or psychological changes that you may be experiencing.

Joan realized that much of her stress was being caused by the fear that, during an office visit, her doctor would tell her that she was going to need joint replacement surgery. Joan's stress reaction—nausea and a tightening of the throat—would appear whenever she imagined this unpleasant occurrence. So she decided to use stress inoculation to gain control. Repeatedly she imagined herself in the very situation she feared. She visualized the doctor's office. She imagined herself sitting in the chair by the doctor's desk. She actually heard the words she feared. As Joan gradually increased her tolerance of this image, her stress symptoms lessened.

Like Joan, whenever you use stress inoculation to visualize and mentally experience a scene, you'll increase your ability to handle that particular stressor, and your symptoms will decrease. In other words, your body and mind will be "inoculated," allowing you to tolerate that stressor. One added advantage of using this technique is that you will become more aware of exactly when these tension-producing situations begin to affect you. This will enable you to use your coping strategies sooner, before your body and mind begin suffering from the stress response.

But don't feel that you have to use stress inoculation for every stressor you anticipate experiencing. And don't think you have to deal with every stressor all at once. Work with each scene individually until you feel you've mastered it.

If you have already read the explanation of systematic desensitization found in Chapter 15, you may realize that stress inoculation and desensitization are very similar. But there is a difference. In desensitization, the technique of imagining a stressful situation is alternated with the use of relaxation techniques. In stress inoculation, relaxation techniques are employed only at the start of each session. Experimentation will show you which method is best for you.

You may also benefit from a "real-life" stress inoculation simply by listening to the stories of others with OA. By learning what others have gone through, in support groups, chat rooms, books, or contact networks, you may become desensitized to some of the issues you may face having OA.

USE PHYSICAL STRESS RELIEVERS

Certain physical activities can be a great means of stress control. For example, some people relieve tension or stress by driving or gardening. As long as you are physically able—and enjoy these activities—either can be very relaxing. But if these aren't your ideas of calming pastimes, there are a number of other activities that may be just the ticket.

Exercise

Exercise is not only a wonderful means of releasing stress but, as we saw in Chapter 9, can be a very healthy component of any treatment program. Regardless of how OA is affecting you, there is certain to be a type of exercise that will help you control your level of stress. Virtually any type of exercise can be effective. Anything that gets the body moving, gets the heart pumping faster, and releases tension is ideal. If you have any concerns about certain activities, just be sure to get your doctor's approval before beginning.

Keep Busy the Fun Way

Hobbies and other leisure activities are often very effective ways to reduce stress. They can divert your attention from the unpleasant situation and direct it toward something more enjoyable. They may also cause you to feel productive—and a lack of productivity may be one of the stressors giving you problems in the first place! If you don't have a hobby, this is a great time to look into one that suits your fancy. If you already participate in leisure activities, now you have the perfect reason to indulge yourself whenever you can.

Catch Up on Your Sleep

Another technique for dealing with stress is sleep. Some people have difficulty sleeping when they're experiencing high levels of stress. But, when possible, catnaps or even prolonged periods of sleep may help you reduce stress to a more manageable level. After all, you need your rest anyway.

A Stress-Free Summary

What are your goals? Are you trying to gain greater control over your emotions? Do you want to live life more fully? Whatever they are, if stress is keeping you from reaching them, then your stress response is negative. By learning how to control your stress—by eliminating the things that are putting pressure on you, or by modifying your reaction—you'll be far more likely to meet these goals. Just as important, you'll have a head start in coping successfully with osteoarthritis.

CHAPTER NINETEEN

Other Emotions

The emotions discussed so far in this section are not the only ones you may experience as a result of your OA, of course. Worry, for example is a basic emotion. What might you worry about? Have you got a month to discuss all the possibilities? You've probably worried about the future, what your life will be like, whether you should have a joint replaced, how life will change because of osteoarthritis, among countless other things. What other feelings could concern you? This chapter will discuss four additional emotions that many people with OA have found to be problematic: boredom, envy, loneliness, and grief.

Boredom

Hopefully, by this time, you are not so bored that you have stopped reading. As long as you aren't bored, let's talk a little bit about boredom.

What an empty feeling boredom is! It's one of the worst feelings you can possibly experience. It has been said that more problems and tragedies are caused by boredom than by any other single emotion. I bet you never thought of OA as being boring. But it can be, primarily because of the restrictions your condition may impose on you. Many activities that provided enjoyment for you in the past may now be out of reach. You may not even want to bother starting something new, as you may feel that future activities will become too restricted due to your condition.

Olive hated the fact that her condition prevented her from knitting. She was tired of music, and she didn't want to read. Was Olive bored? Definitely! But did she have to be? No! Her family and friends suggested new activities for her to try, and Olive soon was able to feel less bored.

So what should you do? To begin with, don't let your condition cause you to give up on life. Distinguish between what you can do and what you can't. If you do have to curtail some activities because of OA, you will do so. If you have to drop an activity, you'll drop it. But don't eliminate all activities simply because you feel that you may not be able to complete them. There are still certain things that hold your attention from time to time, right? How else can you fight the boredom blues? Read on!

TRY NEW ACTIVITIES

If boredom is a problem, the first step is to analyze why you are bored. Obviously, figuring this out will help you determine how you can improve things. Then you'll certainly want to find ways to add some interest to your life. You may find that the activities you used to enjoy now seem artificial and uninteresting. Or that you no longer derive any pleasure from them. Don't feel that you must push yourself to enjoy these activities, as forcing yourself to be amused rarely works. Instead, try to find something new that will make your life more interesting. Remember that preferences change. Be open-minded, and try hobbies, sports, travel, or events that never appealed to you before. This time around, they may spark your interest.

LEARN SOMETHING NEW

One of the most effective weapons against boredom is learning. The mind is like a sponge, always thirsty to soak up information and knowledge. Select a potentially interesting topic that you don't know much about. Then go out and learn something about it. You may want to begin by simply going to the library and reading some books on the topic. Or surf the Internet and see what you can find. Perhaps you'd like to enroll in an adult education course. Boredom often disappears once you become involved in something new. As an added benefit, your new pursuit may put you in contact with some interesting new people. And increasing your circle of friends is always a good way to fight boredom.

SET GOALS

Boredom often arises from plodding along with no purpose in life. So one of the best ways to fight it is to always give yourself something to look forward to—a goal. This doesn't mean that you'll never be bored. You may still have to give yourself an occasional kick in the butt (if your leg or hip doesn't hurt too much) to get yourself moving toward those goals. But the promise of some pleasurable activity will make it much easier to keep yourself going.

What kinds of goals might you set? They can be as simple as reading a chapter of a good book, writing a letter, making that phone call you've been thinking about, watching a television program you've been excited about, or meeting somebody special for lunch. Try to schedule something that will interest you every day. This way, even if part of your day seems boring—because you're involved in more mundane tasks, or because you have to rest to build up your strength—you will at least have something enjoyable to look forward to. You won't give the weeds of boredom a chance to take root!

Envy

You've heard the cliché "The grass is always greener . . ." If you have OA, you're probably envious of those who don't—of people who are fine and don't experience pain, as you do. You may even be envious of other people's joints! This is understandable. But envy is still a destructive emotion, because it's a type of self-torture. When you feel envious, you're constantly putting yourself down and comparing your own qualities with the seemingly better qualities of somebody else. You feel inferior. And this can lead to other negative emotions, such as anger or depression.

Envy is often irrational. When you're envious, you want to be like somebody else. You want to have what somebody else has. Does this mean that the other person has a life that's happier than yours in every way? Stop and think for a moment. I'm sure you can come up with some areas in which your life is better!

IS ENVY A POSITIVE EMOTION?

In general, emotions usually serve a purpose. Emotions such as anger and anxiety mobilize you to prepare to handle their sources. On the other hand, envy is a destructive emotion. It does not have the positive qualities that other emotions have. But maybe you can find something positive in envy. If you recognize that you're envious, analyze the reason why. Try to change your attitude by concentrating on yourself and your own attributes. Don't let envy get you down.

WHAT LEADS TO ENVY?

Basically, there are four conditions necessary for envy to occur. First, you must feel deprived in some way. You must feel as if you can't have something that you want or need. We're not talking simply about money, pleasure, or even health. Envy is an intense emotion that involves much more than this. It seems as if your feeling of need lies deep inside.

Second, to experience envy, you must feel that another person has something you don't have. Perhaps that person has a bigger house, for instance. Or in the case of a person who does not have OA, he or she has good joints.

Third, you must feel powerless to do anything about this problem. You must think that you are unable to change the circumstances that have made you envious in the first place. This helplessness causes you to become more and more bitter. And this makes you even more envious.

Fourth, there must be a change in the relationship between you and the person whom you envy. You are no longer simply comparing yourself with that person; you are now fiercely competitive. You may begin to feel that the only reason you don't have what you want is that somebody else has it.

There are two categories of things that may cause you to feel envy. One is tangible—jewelry, cars, homes, and so on. The other type is less tangible—friends, pleasure, or health, for instance. Even though you have OA, you may still have many tangible things, such as a car and a nice place to live. You may have a good job. But your medical condition can certainly cause you to feel envious over less tangible things.

MAKE THE BEST OF WHAT YOU HAVE

To rid yourself of this destructive emotion, concentrate on increasing those benefits and pleasures you *can* get out of life. Why worry about comparing yourself with somebody else? How is that going to help you? Sure, your body may not be functioning the way it used to. But that doesn't mean you can't get a lot of enjoyment from life. Set up reasonable goals for yourself, considering what valuable things you *do* have and what you are capable of doing. Remember that you are who you are. Make the best of what your life has to offer.

Loneliness

There is a difference between being alone and being lonely. Being alone simply means that there is no one else with you. This can be either good or bad. But being lonely is virtually always a negative. Loneliness is a sad, empty feeling. If you feel lonely, it doesn't really matter whether there's anyone with you. You become upset by your awareness of being alone.

WHY ARE YOU LONELY?

Why might you feel lonely? If you can't spend time with others like you used to as a result of your pain, you may feel left out. Or you may feel lonely because you think that others don't want to be with you, or don't understand your condition. Because you have OA, you may feel isolated from other people who are healthy. And you may decide to change some of your relationships just because you're having difficulty dealing with people.

It's hard to be lonely—and not just because loneliness is such an awful feeling. You see, loneliness doesn't just happen. It actually takes effort to make and keep yourself lonely. There are many opportunities to enjoy the company of others. As a result, loneliness usually occurs out of choice rather than accident. To be really lonely, you must purposely exclude everyone around you from your life. You have to always be on your guard, protecting yourself from the horrible possibility of making new friends!

DO YOU *WANT* TO BE LONELY?

Why would you want to be lonely? There are four possible reasons. First, deep down you may actually enjoy this feeling. In fact, you may enjoy it so much that you refuse to do anything about it. This may contradict your complaints to everyone else. Why might you feel this way? Because you may feel more comfortable alone than in the company of others.

Second, if you're lonely, you may be hard to please. You may feel that you don't want to even bother trying to create new relationships because no one meets all of your requirements.

Third, you may be lonely because you feel that you must be lonely. You may have resigned yourself to it. You may be telling yourself that this is an unavoidable situation due to your OA.

Fourth, and probably most important, you may be lonely because you're scared. You may be afraid of rejection. You may recall previous relationships that didn't work out the way you wanted, and feel that they are simply not worth the hurt and pain.

END YOUR LONELY WAYS

Fortunately, whether your loneliness has been plaguing you for some time or is a relatively new problem, there is a light at the end of the tunnel. Recognize what causes your feeling of loneliness. Admit to yourself that you should try to change this destructive emotion. Then do all you can to fight it.

Don't Be a Pusher

The first step in ending loneliness is to stop pushing people away. It's likely that you're giving off unseen vibrations—vibrations telling people that you don't want them around. These vibrations can reduce your number of acquaintances, adding to your feeling of loneliness. This must stop. You have to learn to give off positive vibrations—the type that welcomes others instead of chasing them away. Smile at people. Show interest in what they have to say and let them know that you like being with them.

Make Contact!

Once you start giving off new, more positive vibes, you'll want to make more friends. How can you meet people? One way is by getting involved in some kind of club or organization. For example, because you have OA, you may want to contact your local chapter of the Arthritis Foundation or other local support programs. There, you'll meet other people with similar concerns. Besides relieving your loneliness, the members of your group may also share some valuable coping skills. You may even find ways of helping others.

If support groups aren't your cup of tea, try getting involved in a new learning activity or hobby. Take adult education courses, for example. This may help to alleviate loneliness as well as boredom. Invite people to your home. (But be sure to pace yourself so that you don't become exhausted.) Most important, be receptive to the people you meet. Try to see the good in everyone. Don't reject someone simply because there are a few things about them that you don't like. (After all, you wouldn't want them to do that to you.)

If you work at conquering loneliness, you'll feel much better about yourself and your life. This will make living more enjoyable, even with OA. Give yourself and others a chance, and your feelings of loneliness will disappear, regardless of the limitations your condition has placed on you.

Grief

Grief is an unpleasant emotion. And feelings of grief—the mourning over a loss—are common in people who have been diagnosed with OA, especially at the time of initial diagnosis or after joint replacement surgery.

WHY ARE YOU GRIEVING?

People grieve when they're aware that they've lost something of value. Although you may never have consciously thought about how much you valued your joints, you may now. OA can make you feel that you have changed or that you have lost some physical strength. As a result, you may not like yourself as much, and are grieving the loss of your self-esteem. If you are used to playing a certain role within your family, and this has been modified due to your OA, you may grieve this loss, as well.

Alice was upset. A 55-year-old mother of three, she had just completed her latest shopping trip and was about to relax in front of her favorite soap opera. She had a gnawing feeling that things just weren't right—she couldn't enjoy her program. My goodness, she had been hooked on this show for almost twenty years! But she decided to turn off the TV and figure out what was upsetting her. After at least four commercials' worth of thought, she realized that it was her soap opera that was bothering her! She felt that the characters on the program, despite all of the script problems, were better off than she was. None of them seemed to be experiencing the pain of OA—only she was! None of them needed medication—only she did! None of them needed daily exercises to keep their joints limber. But she did! As she thought about it, she began to cry. She felt she had lost something from her life, and she was grieving this change.

But grief is not always bad. When this feeling develops, it means that you must work it out before you can adjust to the new situation—in this case, OA.

WORK THROUGH YOUR GRIEF

What can you do about grief? Unfortunately, it cannot be avoided. Only by analyzing your grief and working through it will you be able to get back to the act of living. Alice had to remind herself that actors and actresses have their own problems. She had OA—something she needed to learn to live with. Medication and exercise were keeping her condition in check. She might not like it, but she needed it. She quickly noticed that she was feeling much better. In fact, she was able to turn on the television and enjoy the last few minutes of her show.

How else can you combat grief? Crying can be helpful. This doesn't mean that you should force yourself to sob, but if the tears start welling up, don't stop them. Let your feelings out. Think about what has changed and what will change. Talk it out with the people you trust. Don't avoid the fact that you have OA, as this denial will prevent you from going through the grief process.

Remember that grief is like a deep infection. The only way it can improve is to open it and let what's inside come out, even if it means a good cry. This may be difficult, but eventually the wound will drain and begin to heal. Soon you will exhaust your grief. Then the healing will begin.

Living with OA can involve a number of painful emotions. But it is possible to cope with these emotions—to learn constructive approaches that will eliminate or lessen them, and help you live more comfortably and happily. These strategies are just what the doctor—and family and friends—ordered!

PART FOUR

Interacting with Other People

CHAPTER TWENTY

Coping with Others: An Introduction

You do not live your life alone (unless you're reading this book on a deserted island in the Pacific). You interact with many people every day. So you will certainly want to be able to deal with any difficulties you are having in your interpersonal relationships. For example, you might be worried about what others are going to think about your OA. How are they going to react? Are the going to ask questions? Which answers will help them to understand what you are experiencing, and which ones will turn them away?

Obviously, different problems exist in different relationships. But before we begin discussing all the various people who may be part of your life, here a few general guidelines that you may find helpful.

Do Unto Others . . .

When you interact with others, try not to be too focused on your own feelings. Disregarding the feelings of others will prevent them from getting close to you. So make a conscious effort to be considerate of others, just as you'd like them to consider your feelings.

What does this mean? Just this: *You're not the only one who has to cope with OA*. The important people in your life may also be having a hard time, simply because you mean a lot to them. Remember that. You might not realize that your problems affect those around you. You might think, "Why would they feel upset? It's happening to *me*!" But if you give this some thought, you'll see that you're not being reasonable or fair.

Take your family, for example. A problem for you is also a problem for them. Of course, it may affect you in a different way. You may be the one experiencing the restrictions and the physical changes, as well as the apprehensions and anxieties. But your family doesn't like to see you suffer. In fact, this may explain why family members and friends might be unable to provide all of the support you want as quickly as you want it. Like you, they are probably going through their own period of adjustment.

Then again, rather than being unaware of the emotions of others, you may feel guilty about the added burden you are placing on your family. It can be difficult to cope with this feeling. Keep in mind, though, that you may be projecting this attitude onto your loved ones—and possibly adding to their problems in the process. Chances are, they don't feel as burdened as you may fear. They may feel temporarily helpless or overwhelmed, but still be eager to help.

Change Yourself, Not Others

Do you feel that if you try hard enough, you'll be able to change the attitudes, feelings, or behaviors of others? Unfortunately, it doesn't work that way. Whether the people in your life accept your osteoarthritis or deny that you have any problem at all, you may have a problem changing their thinking. So it makes sense to use your energy to change the one person over whom you do have control—yourself. Spend more time working on yourself, and less time worrying about others. In fact, once others see the changes in you, they may even alter their own attitudes. So help yourself. Be your own best friend.

Look Through the Eyes of Others

If you have an argument with someone, you may believe that you're right and the other person is wrong. If this continues, nothing will be resolved, and the other person's behavior may drive you crazy because it seems so unreasonable.

Take a moment and look at the situation through the eyes of the other person. What does he or she see? What is that person's point of view? Once you've done this, you'll be better able to explain how you feel in a way that he or she will understand. And then you'll be better able to find a solution to almost any problem that might exist.

Learn to Say No

What happens if you're feeling rotten but others want you to keep doing more and more? In the past, you may have had trouble saying no—because you felt guilty, perhaps, or because you wanted to avoid disappointing the other person or hurting his or her feelings. But now things are a little different, and you really must curtail your generosity for the sake of your own well-being. Yes, this may give you the appearance of being selfish. But as long as you don't abuse it, this selfishness can be positive for you. Think of yourself for a change. Only if you take care of yourself will you be able to deal with others. The reverse does not necessarily hold true. If you always take care of others first, this may actually make you less able to care for yourself.

Develop a Strong Support System

You'll find it far easier to deal with OA if you can rely on those closest to you, such as your spouse, partner, other family members, and close friends. This social network can give you added strength in dealing with this disease.

However, it's up to you to decide how to discuss your OA with others. With many medical conditions no one ever needs to be the wiser, although is there really something wrong with people knowing you have this disease? There's nothing to be ashamed of. OA is part of you, just as the color of your hair or eyes is part of you. In addition, there may be a time that you experience an OA-related problem and you need somebody to understand it so that they can help you.

Another advantage to telling people about OA is that you won't feel different when you are with others. They'll view you as simply being a member of their circle of friends, relatives, or acquaintances just as they always have. Also, there may be times when you need encouragement. When people know the problems associated with OA, this encouragement is much easier to obtain.

If you decide that you want to start being more open about OA, determine whom you want to talk to, what you're going to say, and how you're going to say it. You don't have to go into extended detail. You don't have to provide more information than they need or want. Showing how well you're coping will help them to handle it.

Open the Lines of Communication

We've just discussed how the support and understanding of others can help you deal with your OA-related problems. But right now you may find it difficult to even talk to others. So how can you possibly ask for their support? Well, your first job is to open the lines of communication. And how can you do that? The best way to get the conversation rolling is to be open and honest about the way you feel. If you say anything that upsets or hurts somebody else, you'll deal with it then. But first, get your feelings out.

Perhaps you're waiting for others to approach you and offer their support. But since you're the one with OA, you may have to be the first person to talk about it. Other people may be reluctant to even mention the word in front of you. But if you bring it up and talk about it matter-of-factly, you may pave the way to very effective communication.

What if you're too fearful to share your feelings? Certainly, fear can make communication difficult, if not impossible. But don't feel that you have to be too open and talk too much about OA. You don't want it to get to the point where people are tired of hearing about your experiences with this disease.

If, after all is said and done, you find that you don't have the kind of social network that you would like to have, it may be helpful to get involved in a support group. There you will meet people who can provide the caring and understanding you need to cope with OA. (For more information on support groups, see Chapter 12.)

Bring on the World

Now that I've introduced some general ideas, let's see how OA can affect the different relationships that may be part of your life. Of course, not every chapter in this part of the book will apply to you. You may choose to read only those that are appropriate for you, or you may decide to read them all of then. However you choose to approach this material, you'll soon realize that problems exist in all relationships, and there are things that can be done to cope with them successfully.

CHAPTER TWENTY-ONE

Your Family

Blood is thicker than water. Your family can be a critical factor in dealing successfully with OA. Why? You're probably with your family more than with anyone else. If you get along well with members of your family, you'll have a solid foundation from which to move toward a triumphant adjustment to your condition.

Family members may experience many of the same emotional reactions that you do—from anger and depression to worry and frustration. Sometimes family members react more strongly (and possibly less rationally) than the person who's suffering from OA.

Any communication problems that exist within a family may be magnified by the existence of a medical problem. The fact that each person adjusts differently—and may find it hard to change—can also exacerbate family problems.

If you find it difficult to talk to loved ones about your OA, treatment issues, or your feelings, don't give up. To maintain family unity—and to make sure you get the support you need—it is important to bring your concerns out into the open. This doesn't mean that all conversations are going to be pleasant. However, they should enable each person to share his or her feelings with the other members of the family.

Of course, problems may be different for each family member. So let's discuss how you can better deal with your partner, your children, and your parents.

Dealing with Your Partner

Of course, your relationship with your spouse or significant other will be affected by your OA. But this doesn't mean that problems can't be resolved. Better communication, understanding, and counseling (if necessary) can help to resolve most issues. Let's discuss some of the ways OA may affect your primary relationship, as well as various suggestions to lessen its impact.

CHANGES IN YOUR SOCIAL LIFE

Has OA forced you to cut back on some of the social activities you used to enjoy with your partner? There may be times when you are limited due to pain, fatigue, or other symptoms. Although this may be temporary, it can be hard to take, especially if you and your partner have enjoyed active social lives. The partner who does not have OA may feel angry, frustrated, helpless, or bored. You, on the other hand, may feel that you're a burden on your partner. Or you may be angered by what you feel is that person's inability to accept any new restrictions.

Once you have your pain or other problematic symptoms under control, you'll probably be able to resume many of your usual activities. Until then, try to limit yourself to those that require minimal physical energy.

If, however, your social life is still on hold even after you've begun treatment, you will have to ask yourself if this is due to fear, depression, or other emotions. If so, be sure to refer to the appropriate chapters on coping.

IF FAMILY RESPONSIBILITIES MUST CHANGE

What happens if OA creates the need for temporary or permanent changes in each family member's responsibilities? For example, what if it's necessary for your partner, children, or another loved one to take over some of the functions that you performed in the past? This can surely be another potential source of friction between you and that person.

Pat, a 52-year-old homemaker, used to make lunch for her husband and children each morning. But with OA, she was just too stiff early in the morning, and was no longer able to do this. So she transferred this responsibility to her husband. Since he had difficulty boiling water, he wasn't happy about his new assignment. He, in turn, placed added responsibilities on their teenage children. This created even more tension. Despite the fact that Pat's husband and children loved her and were concerned about her health, they were all understandably upset, especially her husband.

How can you make changes as smoothly as possible, without causing your partner unnecessary distress? First, make the changes gradually. Try to avoid overwhelming any family member. And be realistic in your expectations, keeping in mind that it takes time for *anyone* to comfortably incorporate new responsibilities into the normal routine.

How else can you help your partner to adjust to greater burdens? Make sure free time is still available for the pleasures of life. It's only when the new responsibilities seem to be all-consuming that serious problems occur. Be sure to look at any changes through the eyes of your partner. Consider how you'd feel if the situation were reversed. Think how upsetting it would be if you no longer had time for the things you enjoyed because of added responsibilities and pressures. Discuss changes reasonably, and be gentle. Just as important, as these changes occur, be gentle with yourself. When you see other members of your family taking over certain responsibilities, you may feel more and more hopeless and worthless. Look at this as only a temporary situation.

IF YOUR PARTNER DENIES YOUR CONDITION

What can you do if your partner simply won't accept the fact that you have OA? You might hear, "Oh, come on, you don't seem to be in that much pain. What are you complaining about?" Your partner's misconceptions may be tough to swallow. You can, of course, try to educate him or her, but don't go overboard. If you're constantly badgering your partner, pointing out how things must change because of your condition, it may only cause further denial. Keep in mind that your partner will not accept your condition until he or she is ready to do so. In the meantime, concentrate on improving your own thoughts and feelings. Others' feelings may change, but they will do so slowly, and probably not at your urgings.

WHAT ABOUT MONEY?

Osteoarthritis can present added money problems, especially if you handled the family finances and your partner must now share or take charge of financial responsibilities. But even if your partner has always managed the family's money matters, medical bills—and possibly a newly reduced income—can make things tough. Both of you may worry whether you can meet all of your obligations now and in the months to come. Of course, money concerns are a source of friction in many relationships. Here, though, the problem is compounded.

What can you do? Sit down with your partner and talk over your financial situation. Try to be realistic and to reach practical solutions. Admit that new problems may arise, but emphasize the fact that they frequently have a way of getting solved. If not, you will deal with them as they arise. Be patient, be communicative, and, above all, be positive. (For tips on dealing with financial problems, see Chapter 11.)

HAS YOUR SEX LIFE BEEN AFFECTED?

As you may already know, OA can affect sexual relations. If this is a problem for you and your partner, or if you'd just like to learn more about the possible impact that OA can have on sex, see Chapter 25. There you will learn how to solve some of these problems so that sex can remain an important and pleasurable part of your life.

IN SICKNESS AND IN HEALTH? SORRY!

Unfortunately, some relationships have ended because of chronic medical problems. OA-related restrictions, fears, symptoms, and side effects certainly have the potential to drive a wedge into what may have previously been a good relationship, replacing feelings of closeness and intimacy with coldness and distance. This can wash the magic right out of a relationship.

What should you do if your partner is frightened and "wants out"? First, be aware that certain problems may not be entirely your partner's fault. For instance, you may be too apprehensive to enjoy your relationship, so that your problems may be creating a horrible package of anxiety, depression, hopelessness, and panic. What should you do after you try to view things objectively? Get help. This package isn't one you can—or should—handle alone. If communication has become a problem in your home, you may not be able to talk to your partner. The aid of a trained professional or an objective outsider may help to resolve some of the problems that the two of you have been unable to work out yourselves. If possible, include your mate in your counseling sessions. But once again, don't force the issue. If your partner doesn't seem open to outside help, get some counseling for yourself. Regardless of the results of your efforts to save your relationship, any support you can muster will only improve your emotional well-being.

A MARITAL (CON)SUMMATION

Every relationship has its ups and downs, with problems that have to be solved. And OA may make relationships even more vulnerable to crises and arguments. In fact, at some point it may seem very difficult, or even impossible, to deal with your partner. But by giving added attention to your partner's feelings and needs, you will find that many—if not all—of these problems can be resolved over time. And isn't your relationship worth the added effort? Once the two of you address your concerns and make some adjustments, your partner may become your greatest ally in dealing with your condition.

Dealing with Your Children

Children, regardless of how old they are, need a lot of attention, help, and love from their parents. OA can surely be frustrating for everyone if it makes you unable to spend as much time with them as you would like, or if you can no longer do as much for them. This does not mean that you don't love them or that you're not a good parent. You know that. Use the time you do spend with them as productively as possible, and work to help your children handle any fears or changes that may be bothering them. How? Let's see how you can work with your children and help them better cope with your condition.

FOCUS ON QUALITY, NOT QUANTITY

OA can be restricting. Pain, fatigue, medication side effects, surgery— these and many other factors may prevent you from doing a lot of what you'd like to do. Yet you may want to spend as much time as possible with your children. How can you solve this dilemma? You (and your children) must face the reality of your condition. You did not choose to have OA. Honestly explain to your children that you may not always have the strength for certain activities. Then come to an agreement with them regarding some enjoyable things that you can do together when you're feeling better. This arrangement will show your children that you're aware of their unhappiness, and that you do want to spend more time with them.

Also, try to be less concerned with *quantity*—the number of minutes and hours you spend with your kids—and more concerned with *quality*— special time during which you share feelings and pleasurable activities. If your time together is well spent, with plenty of talking and laughing, it will make up for what is missed. And as you share your thoughts with your children, you'll be helping them to better handle any restrictions that result from your OA. Children, especially older ones, can read most of what has been written for adults. They can ask questions, too!

ADOLESCENTS

During adolescence, children begin to assert their independence. Look out, world, the future generation is coming! Adolescents want to start moving away from the family setting and its responsibilities. Even under normal circumstances, this creates problems in many homes. Add a parent with OA to the picture, and the problem is compounded. Why? Because of your condition, your teen may have to help out more than usual around the house. At the same time, your child probably *wants* to do less around the house, and be away more. How can you cope with this predicament? Well, regardless of how much you are truly able to change your teen, perhaps you can learn to cope in a way that, at the very least, keeps you sane. Let's learn more about dealing with adolescents.

Don't Expect Miracles!

First, realize that dealing with teens is quite different from dealing with younger children—which you probably already know. Teens are far more absorbed in themselves than in their families. Remember that they are making quite a few difficult adjustments of their own, and seem to have little interest in others—especially their parents! Of course, not all teens are alike. Some are less self-centered and more sensitive and compassionate than others. Certainly, you know your child better than anyone. But perhaps you now expect your usually insensitive child to rise to the occasion and enthusiastically pitch in with household chores. Be aware that you are probably setting yourself up for disappointment if you expect your child to change so significantly.

Of course, this doesn't mean that you and your teen shouldn't discuss your OA and any limitations you are experiencing. Talk to your child candidly, as you would speak to an adult, as this will probably provide the best chance for a positive response. Think about the concerns your adolescent might have regarding OA, and try to be reassuring. If your teen feels comfortable talking to you about your condition, encourage discussion. But remember to respect the rights of those adolescents who would rather not talk about your illness. And again, don't expect miracles, and don't become devastated if your teenager shows little interest.

When You Need Your Teen to Pitch In

Because of your condition, your adolescent may now have to shoulder more responsibilities. But will your teen be willing to help out? That's the real question!

Sixteen-year-old Jennifer, whose mother had been diagnosed with OA, felt guilty about not helping more at home. However, she thought that giving in would be a sign of weakness. (Heaven forbid!) This caused Jennifer a lot of anguish—which, of course, she didn't want to discuss with her mom. Because of the guilt she was experiencing, Jennifer escaped by spending even more time than usual out of the house—and less time supporting her mother. Jennifer's mom sat down with her, and together they worked out a compromise. Jennifer would not have to spend long hours assisting with chores, but she would make herself available when necessary. After reaching an agreement, both Jennifer and her mom felt closer to each other—and Jennifer felt a good deal better about herself.

So, you see, it may pay to take the initiative and offer a reasonable compromise. Just showing that you understand your teen's feelings may help. Perhaps things won't seem so hopeless to your child, after all.

Another tactic, too, may prove helpful. If your teen must take on some adult chores, consider offering a few adult privileges and pleasures—within reason, of course. Adolescents will usually be more willing to help out if they know that they will be treated and trusted in a more adult way.

Remember that you can go only so far in trying to get your teenager's cooperation. You can't move mountains. Continue to be as constructive as you can, putting on as little pressure as possible in order to keep the door open to good relations. As long as you know you've tried, you can hold your head up high.

Dealing with Your Parents

Parents often have difficulty coping with a child's illness—even if their "child" is an adult. Therefore, if your parents are alive, anticipate that they'll have a rough time. This, of course, will make coping harder for you, too. Why? You don't want your parents to suffer or be upset. And you know how your parents feel, because you'd certainly be upset if any child of yours were ill.

If you have a healthy relationship with your parents, then you're among the lucky ones. But what if you normally have difficulty dealing with them? Having OA won't help! Regardless of the nature of your relationship, consider how your parents have treated you since your diagnosis. Have they ignored or minimized your condition? Or have they smothered you? Let's look at these two possible reactions and see how you can better cope with your parents.

THE IGNORERS

Since Janet's diagnosis with OA two years earlier, her parents had shown less and less concern about her condition. Whenever Janet mentioned that she had pain, her mother told her to just "call the doctor." When Janet was tired, her father told her that "staying in bed won't accomplish anything." Other than making these insensitive remarks, Janet's parents had little to say on the subject of her OA. They certainly never asked questions about her condition. Even worse, when she did try to fill them in, they showed no interest at all.

Parents who ignore or play down your medical condition often do so because they can't deal with it. They don't want to face the fact that their child is sick. (And it doesn't matter how old you are!) Worse, many parents agonize over the possibility that your problem might have something to do with them. While this may not make any sense to you, your parents may be afraid that they did something to contribute to your illness, or that you inherited the condition from them. To avoid these intolerable thoughts, they may try to deny that you have OA, or they may minimize your illness, hoping it will all go away.

Remember what we said in the previous chapter about seeing a situation through someone else's eyes? Don't you think that it holds true in this case? As you look through the eyes of your seemingly indifferent parents, you'll probably realize that this is the only way in which they can cope with the situation right now. Yes, their behavior may change over time, but the change will be gradual and not necessarily in response to your urgings.

THE SMOTHERERS

After Betty was told that she had OA, her mother began visiting her on the average of four times a week. This would have been nice, except: (1) Her mother lived forty-five minutes away by car; (2) her mother was 81, had high blood pressure, and needed to minimize stress; and (3) Betty simply did not want to see her so often. You see, Betty was 56 and often disagreed with her mother—especially regarding how much she should do and the amount of rest she should get. Betty certainly felt smothered.

Parents who smother believe that if you have any kind of problem, they must take care of you. Having OA certainly fits this requirement. It doesn't matter what your marital status is, how old you are, or if you can take of yourself. What matters to them is that they are your parents—they are responsible for your welfare. They'll call frequently, asking how you're doing. They'll want to know what they can do to help. They may come over as often as possible to make sure you're okay. Whether they visit or not, they'll - constantly bombard you with questions about your health and activities.

What can you do, short of moving out of town and taking on a new identity? Again, look at yourself—and your condition—through the eyes of your parents. How do you think they feel? They care about you. What do they see? They see a child who needs them! You may not agree with them, but understanding their point of view should help you better communicate with them and more effectively explain how you feel.

WHAT IF TALKING DOESN'T HELP?

If you've talked to your parents and haven't succeeded in modifying their behavior, at least you know you've tried. This alone may help you feel better. What else can you do? Concentrate on helping yourself feel better. If your parents are unhappy with you because you seem to be rejecting their well-meaning intentions, so be it. If they are unhappy with you because you're making it hard for them to ignore your condition, that's fine, too.

By the way, if you're unhappy with parents who are ignorers, you'd probably love them to smother you for a while. And if you don't like smothering parents, the thought of being left alone is probably very appealing. There's rarely a perfect situation or relationship, and no one gets along with everyone all the time. So instead of complaining about your parents' faults, try to look at the positives in their behavior. This may make you feel better, and will certainly help you avoid going crazy over their actions.

HOW MUCH SHOULD YOU TELL YOUR PARENTS?

A common question of people with chronic illnesses concerns how much they should tell their parents about their problem. Have you worried about this, too? First, think about your parents. How do they usually deal with unpleasant situations? Then ask yourself what, precisely, about your OA you want to share with them. Next imagine how they would react to this, and how you would handle their reactions. All these factors will help you decide how much you should tell them.

For instance, you might wish you could share your fears and worries with your parents so they could offer reassurance. It would certainly be nice to know that you don't have to face something unpleasant alone. But what if your parents couldn't readily accept your problems even if they wanted to? It might be worse to tell them things that they couldn't handle. So don't impulsively blurt out your feelings. By spending a little time determining what's best, you will help yourself feel a lot better. You'll probably improve your relationship with your parents, as well.

Finally, keep in mind that it's sometimes easier to talk to one parent than to the other. Consider telling one of them what's bothering you, and letting that parent tell the other. For example, your mother may be able to get through to your father better than you can. This will make things easier for everybody.

A Familial Conclusion

As you learn to cope with OA, your biggest ally—and an important source of emotional support and practical assistance—may be your family. By learning to deal with your family members in the best possible way, you'll not only make things easier for them but also help them to help you cope with the effects of OA.

CHAPTER TWENTY-TWO

Your Friends and Colleagues

Aside from family, you also interact with friends and colleagues on a daily, or nearly daily, basis. Are there any ways in which you can better deal with these important people? Of course!

Dealing with Your Friends

OA can certainly teach you who your real friends are. Those people you thought were close to you may prove to be not so close. And those people you liked but didn't think would be there for you may, in a pinch, prove to be your most supportive allies. And you can always try to meet new friends. In fact, OA may even help this to happen. How? If you join a support group for people with osteoarthritis, you may meet new and interesting people with whom you have much in common.

Before your diagnosis, your relationships with your friends may have been fairly effortless. Unfortunately, OA can change that. You may be surprised—even hurt—by the seeming aloofness of some friends, while others may be *too* supportive. Then, of course, there are the special problems that may crop up because of your condition—activities canceled because of pain, or the need to ask for help. These are problems that can really take a toll on seemingly strong friendships. How can you handle this? Read on.

BE PREPARED FOR DIFFERENT REACTIONS

How have your friends reacted to your OA? How many even know what this disease involves? They may know the name and even think that they understand what it involves. But because they don't experience pain like you do, they may not be able to really comprehend how you feel. Some may want to learn more; some may want to forget what little they already know.

You should be prepared for a variety of reactions. Some friends, for instance, may seem uninterested and distant. Why would a friend seem distant at a time when you need special support? Well, some people may not know what to say to you. Their heads may be filled with doubts and questions. What should they ask? How should they talk to you? Should they even mention your OA? They may not want to run the risk of stirring up unpleasant feelings for you—or for themselves, if they don't know how to respond. Their doubts and fears may cause so much tension that they don't even want to be with you. Of course, some friends may be very supportive—perhaps too supportive! There may be times when friends keep asking you how you are, or offering help, when you'd simply like to be left alone.

Certainly, friendships can be hurt or lost because of misunderstandings and uncertainties. Can anything be done to prevent these problems from undermining your friendships, or do you have to be a hermit for the rest of your life? Don't despair. There are things you can do to improve the situation.

Try to establish ground rules with your friends. If you're the kind of person who likes to be asked how you feel and wants friends around you at all times, let your friends know. If you'd rather not be asked about your health, let them know that, too. If your feelings fluctuate—if at times you want to talk about the OA, but at other times prefer not to even think about it—make your friends aware of this. Of course, you should realize that this may be difficult for them because they will have no way of knowing how you feel at any given time. So tell them to simply say what's on their minds. You'll let them know if and when you're having trouble.

Clear up the question marks. You can always give your friends information about OA. And if you tell your friends what your needs and desires are, fewer unknowns will exist. The uneasiness about what to do or say, as well as the fear of saying or doing the wrong thing, will be reduced. Communication will be easier, and you and your friends will feel a great deal closer.

CHANGING PLANS

Don't you love having to change plans with a friend at the last minute because you're in so much pain that you can't even move? Probably not. So you can understand how your friends might feel about it. However, good friends, who understand or at least try to understand what you're going through, will probably be able to accept these last-minute cancellations. You may not always get the understanding you want. But you'll probably find at least one or two friends who will be willing to work on a solution to any problems you may have.

ASKING FOR HELP

As you learn to live with OA, you may occasionally have a need to call on your friends for help. You may need help cleaning the house, getting places, taking care of errands, or purchasing groceries, among other things. Are you becoming more selfish? No—although it may seem that way to you. You'd probably like to be able to do these things yourself, but at times it just may not be possible. The reality is that there are certain things that must be taken care of, and if you can't take care of them yourself, you must ask others to help you. So if you need help, reach out for it. That's better than pushing yourself too hard and suffering the consequences.

If you do need help, figure out whom to ask and what they should do. If your friend Myrna loves gardening, it would probably be best to ask her for help with the rosebushes. If you know that Emma suffers from "supermarketitis," requiring daily therapeutic visits to the local food emporium, then being asked to pick up some groceries shouldn't bother her at all. If Mario has a driving phobia, don't ask him to chauffeur you around. Try to arrange for a proper "fit" when asking for help.

When planning to ask a friend for help, keep in mind that older friendships tend to be stronger and more resilient. Such friends will probably be more receptive when approached for favors. Newer or more casual friends should probably not be burdened as much. Without giving a friendship a chance to become firmly planted on your hook, you may lose your prize fish—a good, long-lasting friendship. Also base your choice on the type of help you need. Aim for a proper fit. (By the way, no matter how old and dear the friend, once you feel up to it, it would be nice to show your appreciation through an unexpected gift or gesture.)

What should you do if your friends complain or show resentment when you request help? Back off for a while. In addition, try to talk it over with them. Discuss these problems when the conflict can still be resolved; don't let them build up until the friendship is destroyed. If your efforts to mend the friendship fail, remember this: Friends who can't understand your need for help are not very good friends anyway.

LOSING FRIENDS

What if it just doesn't work out the way you want? For example, what if the people you thought were your friends don't call or visit? What if they seem reluctant to include you, preferring to "wait and see how you feel"? When friends seem to drift away, it's certainly sad. But remember that it was not your decision to end the friendship. And you don't want it to be your problem!

Why might this have happened? Maybe your friend felt uncomfortable being with you. Maybe he or she was "turned off" by the fact that you have a medical problem. Or perhaps that person was unsure of what to say or do. Whatever the reason, you've probably learned a hard, unpleasant lesson: You can't change someone else's feelings.

A sturdy relationship, even if it has to go through some rough times, will probably end up even stronger than before. There may be times, however, when a friend or lover cannot handle your condition and you feel as if you've been rejected. This can be devastating—especially if you fear that you won't be able to develop any other meaningful relationships. Nonsense! You are still the same person you were before, except for the ways that OA has affected you physically. Keep telling yourself this so you can restore any confidence that may have been shaken by your friend's action. Be reassured that most people who lose friends because of OA do make new ones. Anyway, you really don't want a "friend" who is uncomfortable with you. You want a friend who likes you for who you are—OA and all. And there are plenty of wonderful, understanding people out there. So don't give up!

Dealing with Your Colleagues

If you work, you're probably spending many hours a week with a number of colleagues. These people are likely to show a variety of reactions to your condition (if they know about it), as well as to any impact it might have on your work. Let's discuss some of the ways in which you may better cope with your colleagues.

SHOULD YOU TELL YOUR COLLEAGUES?

Hopefully, if you're comfortable with yourself, others will be, too. Many colleagues will take your condition in stride, and won't even think about it. Might it be helpful to provide them with some basic information on OA? It could be, although you should realize that this will not necessarily improve their attitude toward you or this disease. Unfortunately, knowledge doesn't always lead to understanding. However, just knowing that you've tried to help educate your colleagues might make you feel better.

Of course, unless nosy colleagues ask questions, you may decide not to even bother telling your coworkers about your OA. Obviously, there is no requirement that you do so.

IF COLLEAGUES ARE RESENTFUL

Jack was a 59-year-old salesman who had worked in the same showroom for twenty-nine years. Because of OA, Jack occasionally found it necessary to reduce his ten-hour-a-day work schedule to five hours. This plan was endorsed by his physician and employer, but was not accepted graciously by his colleagues, many of whom would have liked similar arrangements. This caused bitterness and strain between Jack and his colleagues.

If you have to curtail your working hours, or find that you must occasionally miss work because of OA, you, like Jack, may encounter some resentment. At this point, you may decide to explain your situation to your colleagues, or you may prefer to keep this information to yourself. Either way, accept the fact that some people just won't want to understand what's happening to you and why. Remember: You can't change another person. If a colleague—or anybody else, for that matter—can't handle or understand the effects of your disease, that's his or her problem. You can try to educate people about OA, but you shouldn't make their attitude your problem. If you've got an employer with an open mind, you are very fortunate. Don't be as concerned about the attitudes of coworkers. Instead, concentrate on doing what's best for you.

COOPERATIVE COLLEAGUE COMPROMISES

Occasionally, you may find yourself unable to complete all of your work. When this happens, try to make an arrangement with a colleague. What type? Certainly, it depends on the relationship between you and the other person, as well as on the type and amount of work to be done. You might, for instance, offer to pay your coworker for completing your assignment. Or you might offer to perform a task for a coworker at some later date.

This type of arrangement may seem strange—even uncomfortable at first—but it can result in even better relationships between you and your colleagues. You have nothing to lose. The worst thing your coworker can do is say is no.

Whether you need to work or simply enjoy working, you'll certainly want to minimize any potential occupational problems your OA has caused. And you'll certainly want to maintain good friendships so that you can continue to participate in interesting and emotionally supportive social activities.

EMPLOYER ACCEPTANCE OR HARASSMENT?

Let's say that you've been working for a while but your employer has been expressing his displeasure about curtailed work time. What if he or she issues an ultimatum, stating that if productivity does not improve, you will be discharged? This is a potential problem. What should you do? You do the best you can. If an employer doesn't understand enough about OA to know that you must pace yourself and shows little or no willingness to cooperate, then you're probably better off not continuing employment there. You don't want to look for trouble.

For financial reasons, should you wait until your employment is terminated? This idea has its pros and cons. If you receive unemployment benefits for losing your job, this could ease financial burdens. But if subsequent employers are reluctant to hire you because of the grounds for dismissal, is it worth it? Only you can decide, and you'll probably have to base your decision on your own unique situation. It's a very important question, since your psychological state is so important when you cope with OA. If your employment is aggravating you, then changes may have to be made.

Time to Punch Out

Whether dealing with friends or coworkers, always take one day at a time. Don't worry about unforeseen problems that may never occur. If and when your OA does cause a problem, identify it quickly. Then don't hesitate to use the best strategies to resolve the dilemma, and to restore good relations between you and the people you interact with on a daily basis.

CHAPTER TWENTY-THREE

Your Physician

How do you feel about your physician? (What a question!) Some people see physicians as gods. Others feel that they're rich, indifferent, cold professionals who really don't want to help. Of course, there are other opinions. What's your feeling? Your own view of your doctor will help determine how your treatment progresses. You may find that your feelings toward your physician—or toward physicians in general—have changed since your diagnosis. Some people with OA don't have as much confidence in their physicians, figuring that if their problem had been treated differently, maybe their OA would have been better controlled. Let's learn more about the doctor-patient relationship and see how you can work more effectively with your own physician.

Finding the Right Doctor

Many people with OA wonder which type of doctor should be responsible for their treatment. The consensus is that your primary physician should be a board-certified rheumatologist who will—hopefully—be your advocate in determining which treatments are best for you, both now and in the future. Your doctor will also help coordinate the efforts of any other physicians who may be involved in your care. This physician will help you manage your pain, provide guidelines for any lifestyle changes that may be beneficial or necessary, and even work with you when medical problems unrelated to OA occur.

What should you look for when choosing your primary physician—or any physician, for that matter? First, you want someone who is highly qualified to treat osteoarthritis. The reason for this is clear. But just as important, you want someone you're comfortable with personally. You see, research has suggested that the greater your comfort level, the more likely it is that you will comply with prescribed treatment, and the better you may respond to this treatment. And, of course, you must remember that you may have to visit your physician more often than does someone without a chronic medical problem.

Many factors will determine how comfortable you might feel with your physician, including your personality, your doctor's personality, your age, your doctor's age, your doctor's philosophy regarding treatment, and more. Remember that the chemistry between a doctor and each patient is unique. Although a friend or relative may recommend the "perfect" doctor, he or she may not be right for you. So select a physician whom you can trust.

Of course, we all want the perfect doctor—the one with the best credentials, the most experience, the most impressive reputation, and the warmest bedside manner. (And, of course, the office should be right around the corner!) But accept the fact that you probably won't be able to find a doctor who meets all of your criteria. Determine what you feel is the most important. You may, for instance, be willing to accept a doctor with excellent qualifications whose treatment recommendations are your first choice, even if he or she is lacking in bedside manner. Use your best judgment, and make the decision based on those criteria with which you feel the most comfortable.

Creating a Good Doctor-Patient Relationship

Once you've chosen your primary physician—and, possibly, other health-care professionals—you will want to develop a good relationship. There are two fundamental things you can do to help make—and keep—your relationship pleasant and, most important, beneficial.

SET COMMUNICATION GROUND RULES

It's vital to set ground rules regarding communication with your doctor or any health-care professional. In the past, physicians believed that patients with chronic illnesses should be burdened with as little detailed information as possible, so they limited the amount of information they shared. Today, this is not as often the case. Many people with OA want to be actively involved in their treatment and to review all the facts. Regardless of how much information you want, be sure to clearly communicate your needs. Of course, this is a fairly simple matter if you desire as little as possible or want to be told everything. But what if you want your communication to fall somewhere in between? Be aware that there's nothing wrong with saying, "Doctor, I really want all the information about my case. But please remember that I'm very sensitive, so try to tell me things as gently as possible!"

CLARIFY YOUR ROLE IN TREATMENT

At the beginning of a new relationship with any health-care professional, be sure to clearly explain the kind of role you want to play in your own treatment. Some people want to be very actively involved in making treatment decisions. Others want to find a professional they can trust, and then let that person run the show. Either approach is fine, depending on your preferences. Make sure that you not only communicate this, but that your doctor is comfortable with this arrangement. This is vital for a good working relationship that will result in the best outcomes.

You will need to be comfortable discussing different treatment options with your doctor. Take time to read and gather information. Talk to others about their experiences. Then you can select a course of medical treatment or surgery from a place of strength and knowledge.

Getting the Most from Office Visits

Most communication with doctors occurs during office visits. We certainly want these visits to be as helpful and productive as possible. But as you may know, this is sometimes more easily said than done. All of us have probably come home from a doctor's visit and realized that we forgot to ask an important question. Or perhaps we did ask the question, and then promptly forgot the answer. Nothing can be more frustrating—especially since physicians are often difficult to reach by phone. Fortunately, there are ways to avoid this frustration. Let's look at some of the easy things you can do to get the most from your office visits.

MAKE A LIST

Before each appointment, it is important to prepare a list of all the questions you want to ask your doctor. Don't wait until the night before your office visit to do this. Instead, on an ongoing basis, record notes whenever a question or other detail enters your mind.

Although making a list may seem elementary, it is an excellent way to obtain the information you need to better understand your OA, properly care for yourself, and guide your treatment. Don't be concerned that the doctor won't like the idea that you've prepared a list of questions. Most good doctors appreciate this practice because it tends to structure the appointments more efficiently. However, if your doctor doesn't like it, ask yourself this: Whose treatment and condition is on the line, anyway?

Besides those questions that occur to you, you may want to include concerns expressed by family members or close friends—even if you feel that their points may not be important. Your doctor will be able to tell you what is relevant, as well as provide you with the answers.

Many people worry that the questions they have are too simple and trivial, or even foolish. Remember that the only foolish question is the unasked one. If you need further explanation of something related to your OA or a particular treatment, feel free to ask and to be as straightforward as possible. This will make it easier for your doctor to respond with the information you need.

GET THE ANSWERS

As your doctor or other health-care professional answers your questions, be sure to listen carefully. How annoying it is to realize that you've been looking at the next question, rather than listening to the response. If you're worried that you won't remember everything, there are three ways to help your memory. The first is to jot down notes as each question is answered. The second is to bring a tape recorder. The third is to bring a family member or close friend.

Taking someone along is often a good idea, not because you need someone to hold your hand, but because two sets of ears are always better than one. Going to the physician's office can be stressful, so it's easy to miss what's said. In fact, studies have shown that people remember only a fraction of what their doctors tell them during office visits. Having extra listeners will increase the likelihood that you receive all important information, and also relieve some of the pressure, helping you to relax and more efficiently listen and respond. Following the doctor's visit, you and the person who went along can compare notes.

If you do decide to bring a family member or friend with you, tell that person what you want to accomplish during the appointment. Review the questions you want to ask, and the information you hope to obtain. Your family member or friend will then be able to intervene and ask any questions that you may overlook.

If the purpose of your office visit will be to determine surgery options for OA, consider having several people attend with you. This will allow each one to feel involved. Of course, you and your doctor will make the final decision on how you will ultimately proceed.

Feel free to request additional information about any issues your doctor discusses. It is certainly well within your rights to question any aspect of the treatment that is prescribed or recommended, as well as any medication, diagnostic or surgical procedure, or other options. Some people, of course, prefer not to ask questions, but to simply follow the dictates of their physician. This, too, is within your rights. But keep in mind that in a situation in which you want to do everything possible to help yourself, the more you know, the better.

Of course, we all want to have confidence in our doctors—to believe that they are experts in a particular field. This doesn't mean, however, that you must blindly accept everything your doctor says. For the most part, physicians respect patients who ask questions. Don't feel you are powerless to disagree. If you are unsure of the reason behind a recommendation, question it. It's very important to be honest with your physician—as well as with yourself. If you don't like a particular treatment, or if it doesn't seem to be working for you, you have the right—in fact, the obligation—to say so.

It's also important to indicate when you don't understand your doctor's answers because they're either too vague or too technical. Don't hesitate to raise additional questions. Perhaps your physician uses only specialized, scientific terms. Other patients may be too intimidated to ask for clarifications. Whatever the reason for the problem, don't be afraid to talk openly and honestly. And don't be embarrassed. Your goal is to talk more comfortably and intelligently about what's happening to you. If you don't understand something, or if you don't agree with a treatment plan, inform your doctor.

OTHER CONSIDERATIONS

What else can you do to make your office visits as beneficial as possible? Remember that you are the only one who really knows how you feel. If you think that there is something happening that your doctor should know about, be sure to mention it and make sure that you're heard. Don't think that any piece of information is unimportant, even if the doctor doesn't seem to be as impressed by a particular statement as you expected. Every bit of information that you give can and should help your doctor determine the best treatment course for your OA.

Perhaps you're hesitant about giving your doctor all the facts. You might be afraid that you'll be hospitalized if your doctor finds out how you're really feeling. You might be concerned that your physician won't like some of your "bad" habits. You might fear that you'll be labeled as a complainer who's crying wolf, and then won't be taken seriously when an emergency occurs. Or you might worry that your physician will increase your medication—or not increase it. Despite these concerns, you do want your physician to provide the care that is best for you. This is possible only when you're completely open and honest about the way you've been feeling and how you've been caring for yourself.

While you are at the office, also make sure you have a clear understanding of any medication that has been prescribed during the visit. Be certain you know its actions, any foods to eat or avoid with the medication, and any side effects you might expect. (For more information on medication, refer to Chapter 6.)

By the time you leave the doctor's office, you will, hopefully, have had your questions answered and agreed on your treatment program. By all means, follow this program. But be sure to report any problems that may occur during treatment. And don't expect instantaneous results. It can sometimes take weeks for your body to respond to a new treatment.

Knowing When to Contact Your Doctor

One of the most important questions you'll want to ask your doctor is when to call about a problem. Which symptoms should be reported immediately? Which are not as important, and can be reported at the next regular visit? Ideally, you should get this information as early as possible in your relationship. Ask about the specific symptoms, events, side effects, or other problems that you should report, and also ask the best time to call. But when in doubt, check it out. Don't sit by your phone wondering if you should pick it up; just do so. Remember that if you are taking a new med-

ication, you cannot be expected to know exactly how your body will respond. The doctor has been through this many times, and can tell you that
it wasn't necessary to call at this time (and why). After you've lived with a
certain treatment, medication regimen, or some of the effects of OA for a
while, you'll have a better idea of when you should call.

Getting Second Opinions

Because you may not agree with everything your physician says, and because no physician knows everything, you might want a second opinion, or
even a third. It's always important to get additional opinions if you have
been diagnosed with a chronic medical problem, or if the prescribed treatment is aggressive—for instance, if surgery has been recommended. This
does not necessarily mean that you are questioning the initial diagnosis or
prescription for treatment. It simply means that you are wisely exercising
caution and seeking as much information as possible.

Many people worry that if they seek another opinion, they will hurt
their physician's feelings. Are you reluctant to bring up the idea because
you think you will anger the doctor? Keep your chief priority—your own
well-being—in mind, and remember that your doctor is there to treat you
and serve you. *You* are the one who ultimately makes the decisions. In addition, realize that many good physicians will accept—even value—your
desire to get a second opinion. In fact, they may take your decision as a
matter of course. A good physician will recognize that a second opinion
will either confirm what she believes or point out the need for further discussion.

WHOM SHOULD YOU CONTACT?

The physician you contact for a second opinion should certainly have as
much experience as your primary doctor—or more. But how can you get
an appropriate referral? You may start, of course, by asking your family
physician or primary physician for a recommendation. If this doesn't work,
you can check with the Arthritis Foundation, or with the chief or assistant

chief of the department of rheumatology in hospitals in your geographic area. Or you can check with your county or state medical society, which is probably listed in your local telephone book. You might also have to check with your health insurance provider, who can give you a list of physicians whose services are covered by your insurance plan. And, of course, you may wish to seek recommendations from people you know—especially from others who have themselves been treated for OA. Support groups are another good place to learn the names of physicians who specialize in osteoarthritis treatment.

THE SECOND OPINION . . . AND BEYOND

When you go for a second opinion, make sure that you carefully select and prioritize your questions. Keep in mind that you may not have to ask the same basic questions you asked your primary physician when you were first learning about OA treatment options. Remember why you're going for the second opinion, and focus on the information that you wish to obtain. Then let the conversation, as well as your written list of questions, guide you.

If the second opinion significantly differs from the first, you might try to bring the various professionals together to discuss diagnosis and treatment. Physicians often discuss their findings by phone. If this is not possible, however, it may be in your best interest to seek a third opinion. Understandably, you may find this an unappealing option, both because of the pressure it places on you to find another qualified physician and because of financial considerations. Remember, though, that this is your life! So if a third opinion seems to be in order, by all means, get it.

Before we leave the subject of second and third opinions, remember that there is a difference between changing physicians and seeking another opinion. A second opinion serves to validate or question your current doctor's diagnosis or prescribed treatment. Nor am I suggesting that you continually shop around for the "ideal" doctor, as no such person exists. However, a second opinion can give you the information—and peace of mind—you need to select the best way to treat your OA.

You're Not Locked In

Some people have a lot of trouble with the idea of changing physicians. Others seem to change physicians more often than they change their clothes. If you're not happy with your physician, you're not under any obligation to continue seeing him or her. Don't see a particular physician if you feel intimidated about asking questions or calling when there is a problem. It's best to find another physician if you lack confidence in the information you're being given, or in the course of treatment that's being prescribed. Finally, don't continue seeing your physician if you feel that he or she doesn't care about you and doesn't have your best interests at heart.

However, before you begin seeking another doctor, carefully examine the reasons you want to switch. Are you changing because your doctor doesn't give you the appropriate information at the appropriate time? Are you changing because he or she doesn't seem compassionate enough? As much as possible, try to pinpoint the cause of the problem.

After determining what it is that you don't like about your doctor, attempt to decide if your concern is valid. Be aware that from time to time just about all people who are living with the discomfort of OA experience anxiety—anxiety that can spill over into the doctor-patient relationship, causing problems. Add to this the fact that physicians may not always have the answers—may not always be able to reduce pain or alleviate side effects, or to predict the results of a given treatment. Thus, tensions may rise even higher. Is this type of tension affecting your judgment of your doctor? Or is there, in fact, a real problem that must be solved?

If the problem is, in fact, valid, you have three options. Option number one is to continue seeing your doctor under the present (less than desirable) conditions. Option number two is to be more assertive, and to discuss the situation with your doctor in the hopes of improving your relationship. Option number three is to simply change doctors without trying to salvage the relationship.

Obviously, the first option is not a good one. Staying with a doctor who makes you unhappy is not going to contribute to your well-being.

Number two, however, may be worth considering. Many people find that talking to their doctors about their concerns in a constructive, positive way can solve problems. In some cases, it isn't necessary to change doctors. How might you approach your doctor about problems with your relationship? Don't try to do it by phone or at the end of a regular examination. Instead, schedule a separate consultation so that you will have the time to sit down and discuss your concerns. Once your doctor is aware of the problem, you may very well be able to reach a mutually satisfactory solution.

But perhaps you don't feel comfortable approaching your doctor this way. If you are afraid of being honest—or feel that your doctor simply can't provide the care you need—this relationship may not be the one for you. If so, option number three may be the best choice.

If You Need to See Several Doctors

It is possible that, during your treatment for OA, you may need to see additional health-care professionals. But it can be frustrating if no one professional knows all the relevant information about your case. Inevitably, there are communication gaps. Even though some of your physicians may work together and try to keep one another informed, there is always something lost in each communication.

Is this a hopeless situation? Absolutely not! When communication gaps exist, either you or your primary physician can become the intermediary—the one who makes sure that each professional involved has all the necessary information.

First, whenever you are referred to someone for the first time, be sure to contact the offices of your present doctors and request that copies of your records be forwarded to the new physician. Then be sure to take your own personal anecdotal records, dating back to the time you began dealing with your condition. What should you have in your records? Include all relevant information about your symptoms. List every doctor you have seen—along with specialty, address, and telephone number—any diagnoses that have been made, and treatments prescribed. Also include a list of all the diagnostic tests that you've received, dates, and the results. Detail all prescribed treatments, describing the results, including both the benefits and the side effects. Also record any medications prescribed, including the name, dosage, the length of time you took them, and side effects, if any. Any other details you feel are important may, of course, also be included.

Keep on updating this information using a word processor, if possible, so that whenever you see a new doctor, you can quickly produce an easy-to-read copy. As time goes by, this information may prove to be invaluable.

In Conclusion

Your goal in life may not have been to become an expert on OA. Nor is it likely that your goal was to keep ongoing records of your medical history, or to sharpen your communication skills. But you'll find that your efforts in all of these areas will pay big dividends when dealing with doctors—the biggest dividends being greater health, management of symptoms, and better coping skills.

CHAPTER TWENTY-FOUR

Handling Comments from Others

As Ralph Kramden of *The Honeymooners* would say, "Some people have a B-I-G MOUTH!" You may agree with this when you think of some of the comments you hear from people around you. They may be close friends or even relatives, but that doesn't mean they know how to talk to you about osteoarthritis or what you're feeling. They may say things that they feel are true, witty, intelligent, or even sympathetic. But you may think otherwise. There may be times when a comment makes you want to implant your knuckles in the speaker's teeth. Or a comment might make you wonder if you're talking to a graduate of the Ignoramus School of Tactlessness.

As you know by now, you cannot change other people. You cannot make them more sensitive or teach them how to be more tactful. But you *can* learn how to cope with some of the ridiculous comments you may hear.

Are Others Being Cruel?

Before we discuss the techniques that will help you cope with annoying comments—and the annoying people who make them—it's important to recognize that most people say things out of sincere concern. They may be trying to make you feel better, to show their support, or to show an interest in you by asking how you're feeling. Does that mean you must always be receptive to their questions and respond to all of them seriously? Despite the good intentions behind these comments, it may not always be possible to respond to them politely and thoughtfully. The problem is that hearing the same questions over and over can get on your nerves. Initially, you may try to gently respond to comments or questions, or to politely change the subject. But this may not always work.

Certainly, some people with OA avoid unwelcome comments simply by keeping their condition a secret. For the purpose of this chapter, though, let's assume that we're discussing those comments that you can't avoid, made by people who haven't yet learned to tune in to your feelings. If you've never experienced any comments of this nature, that's great! But read on anyway. You never know when a tip might come in handy.

How Should You Respond?

Many of the things that people say to you may be legitimate comments, but may bug you just the same. Others may not even deserve answers. Some people may make remarks without any consideration of your feelings. But it doesn't matter why a comment is inappropriate. What's important is that you handle these comments in a way that makes you feel comfortable.

How might you respond to an annoying comment? There are three ways that might prevent a further stream of remarks, while making you as comfortable as possible. The first way is to ignore the comment. This is not always easy, especially if the person persistently waits for your answer or seems genuinely insulted by your lack of response. How do you get them to stop asking (short of buying a muzzle)? If you are able to change the subject or walk away—in other words, ignore the question—you may get that person to stop asking.

The second way is to answer in a rational and intelligent way, explaining how you feel or what you sincerely want to communicate. This may satisfy the person and stop the remarks or questions. But, of course, there's a limit to the number of times you can explain something, especially if what you're saying isn't being understood or accepted. (And this certainly isn't good for your physical health!)

As you've probably experienced, you may not always be able to ignore a remark or respond in a rational way. So what can you do when these two approaches fail? There's got to be a better way, and there is. You can use humor. Why would this work? Well, if the person's comment is really unanswerable, you're going to have a little fun with your response, and humorously let that person know that the remark may have been somewhat inappropriate. This technique is called *paradoxical intention.* You're responding in a way that's opposite of what the person might expect. Let's use the remainder of the chapter to look at some of the comments you may hear, and see how you can use paradoxical intention to answer the unanswerable—without losing your sanity or saying things that you might later regret.

Handling the "Big Mouth" Syndrome

What might you hear? And how should you handle it? Remember, the best response is one that will educate the commenter. You'd like to explain your situation nicely, in a nonoffensive, sincere way. But you're only human. So how can you respond when you get fed up? Read on. . . .

"YOU LOOK AWFUL!"

It can be very upsetting when somebody says "Wow, do you look lousy!" You may feel lousy, but you certainly don't want to be reminded of it. And you surely don't want to think that the way you feel is so obvious to others. You'd like to believe that you at least look okay to those around you. Even if it's said sympathetically, this remark may be insulting. So what can you say? You might respond, "Thank you, so do you!" Or "Yes, I know. I've worked hard to look that way." Or, if you're really in a cynical mood, you might say, "I know I look lousy. That comes from hearing people tell me I look lousy all the time." Of course, you could always say, "That makes sense, since I don't feel so hot, either."

"WHY DO YOUR FINGERS LOOK LIKE THAT?"

Most considerate people won't ask ridiculous questions such as this. But every now and then, you might encounter someone who is so absorbed with himself or herself that common courtesy is overlooked and curiosity takes over. So what do you do if you don't want to explain how the inflammation of OA has affected your joints? You might say, "My fingers did too much walking through the Yellow Pages." Or "They work better when they look this way." Or "My real name is Pinocchio, but it isn't my nose that grows." Of course, you could put the other person on the spot by asking, "What's wrong with them?" as you smile innocently.

"ARE YOU SURE YOU NEEDED JOINT REPLACEMENT SURGERY?"

What if a friend finds out that you've had a hip replaced and says, "You should have gotten a second opinion. You probably didn't need it." Besides retorting that you did get a second opinion, how else can you respond to this? You might answer by saying, "You're right, I don't need it. I just love being confined to bed." Or else "You're right, I should have gone to more doctors. The smell of the antiseptic excites me!" Or "I decided that I needed it so my leg would be strong enough to help me run away from people who say ridiculous things!"

"WHAT DID YOU DO TO YOURSELF?"

Some people are convinced that whenever something goes wrong, it is a result of personal neglect. You meet a friend in the street who says, "If only you had eaten better, this wouldn't have happened." You could reply, "What should I eat now, a new joint?" If someone asks why you seem tired, you might respond, "Normally I don't seem so tired, but I just finished a marathon dance contest." Or you could say, "I'm tired from kicking people who keep asking me what I did to myself." This doesn't suggest that you be unfeeling in your answers. However, if you need to let the commenter know that you don't appreciate these question, that'll do it.

"GET BUSY!"

You are quietly sitting in a chair because the pain is keeping you from moving comfortably. Somebody comes over to you and asks what's wrong. You try to explain that any movement is increasing your pain so you're trying to move slowly. In a concerned way, the person says, "You're spending too much time thinking about yourself. Just get out of that chair and do something. Soon you won't even remember that you're not feeling well!"

How would you react to that? Would you jump out of your chair? Of course not. If you weren't feeling so much pain, you wouldn't be sitting there in the first place. Would you try to explain that you're feeling terrible? No, because this person is obviously convinced that the pain you're feeling really doesn't matter. You might say, "I would like to get up, but somebody put fast-drying glue on the chair, and I'm stuck forever." Or you might respond, "I'm trying to set a Guinness world record for the most time spent sitting in a chair." Obviously, the type of response you use would depend on how angry or irritated you feel.

Remember: For this approach to work best, you want to keep your tone of voice as light as possible. This will show the person making the comment that you're fine but that you simply don't appreciate what's being said.

"HOW CAN YOU STAND SO MUCH PAIN?"

In response to this profoundly sympathetic expression of curiosity, you might want to ask, "What pain? The pain from my joints or the pain I get from these dumb questions?" Or you might want to point out other feelings, using a remark such as this: "I've grown rather accustomed to not being able to move!" Or you might simply say, "I don't stand it. I usually have to lie down." People will get the message. You may not like the pain of OA, but at least you're learning to cope with it.

"WHAT'S OSTEOARTHRITIS?"

Plenty of people are aware of what arthritis is, even if they don't know that what you've got is called osteoarthritis. But how do you respond if somebody asks what it is, or says "I never heard of OA," and you're tired of explaining? You might say, "Let's forget you even brought it up. Then you can keep your streak going." Or you could say, "I never heard of it either. How's the weather?" Don't forget: You really don't want to hurt the person's feelings by being sarcastic. If the question is a sincere desire for information, then you can provide a simple answer or offer a brochure on the subject. However, coping with comments from others can be one of the hardest things about living with OA. There are times when being gentle and tactful with others is less important than helping yourself to handle comments without becoming aggravated.

Other Lovable Comments

What are some of the other comments that you may hear? How many of the following have come your way?—"Is osteoarthritis contagious?" "How do you get dressed?" "Why don't you quit your job?" "You should exercise more!" "Are you sure you can walk up those stairs?" "Your hands look strange!" "Rest. Don't do anything!" "What did the doctor say?" "How's your hip?" "What is the prognosis?" "Wow, have you changed!" "You must miss the way you used to feel!" "What's the matter with you?" "What does your scar look like now that you've had surgery?" "It could be worse—you could have cancer!" "You can't possibly have that much pain!" "Thank goodness I don't have it!" "That pain is all in your head!" "If you ate right, you'd feel better!" "Why don't you try my doctor?" "I certainly don't envy you!"

Is That All?

It would fill volumes to include all of the comments that you might hear from "well-meaning" friends or relatives. Hopefully, by reading the previous examples, you've gotten a good idea of how you can respond in a humorous way. Perhaps you'll be able to come up with some additional goodies. Remember that you don't want to be sarcastic or cruel. Rather, you want to show the speaker that you're feeling well enough to respond with humor and spirit. And you want to show that you can certainly do without this person's "helpful" bits of information and "words of encouragement."

Perhaps you're thinking, "I could never say those things. It's just not my style." Well, you don't always have to respond this way. But you can at least *think* such comments. Even that may help you feel better. And keep in mind that even if you don't want to use this type of response all the time, it might come in handy occasionally—when it seems appropriate for you. As you learn to respond more comfortably to others' comments, you'll find that you can handle them more calmly. Then you'll be able to minimize the sarcasm, and respond with more humorous and enjoyable answers.

A Final Comment

Remember, the purpose of this chapter is not to prepare you for the Mean Person of the Year Award. Rather, it is to give you additional tools to use when you get frustrated at the comments others make about OA or your symptoms. Increasing your confidence in handling other people is an important goal. You can achieve it by using different techniques like humor, ignoring the individual, offering a brochure, or biting your tongue.

One of the most common and yet most irritating comments that you may hear has been saved for last. Imagine that somebody who is supposedly sympathetic and trying to help you feel better turns to you with eyes full of compassion and concern and says, "I heard about someone who was crippled from osteoarthritis!" As you turn to walk away, you respond, "I heard about someone who was crippled after telling someone with OA what you just told me." You walk away, head held high and a smile on your face, leaving the astonished well-wisher behind you.

CHAPTER TWENTY-FIVE

Your Sex Life

This chapter is *not* rated R, for Restricted. Rather, it is rated E, for Essential. Why? If you are sexually active, you certainly don't want osteoarthritis to prevent you from having an enjoyable sex life.

Has OA decreased your sexual appetite or ability? This can have an important bearing on the closeness of the relationship with your partner. What kind of sexual relationship did you have before you were diagnosed? Was it a solid one, or was it on shaky ground? If you had a good sexual relationship, you'll have an easier time getting over any obstacles that OA may have thrown into your sex life. If your sexual relationship wasn't good, it is unlikely that having OA will make it better. You may need some professional help to keep things from breaking down altogether. And if pain, medication, or surgery has created problems, some adjustments may be necessary. But all hope is not lost. If you unite with your partner to work things out together, reassure each other, relearn how to please each other, and show a desire for each other, in all likelihood you will eventually resume or continue to enjoy pleasurable sex.

Sexual problems related to osteoarthritis can be physical or psychological in origin, or they may be a combination of the two. Let's look at both categories of causes, and explore some coping strategies.

Physical Problems

Can physical problems alter your interest in sex? You bet your hormones they can!

There is no question that OA can have an effect on your sex life. What can cause some of the difficulties? How about pain, stiffness, and fatigue? Not to mention the treatments for these symptoms.

WHAT CAUSES PHYSICAL PROBLEMS?

It's very hard to enjoy sexual activities or even engage in them at all if you're in a lot of pain, or if sex itself becomes painful. This pain can decrease both your desire and your ability to participate in sex. Most sexual problems are mechanical, related to pain and joint restrictions, since the genitals are not directly affected by osteoarthritis. Many people with OA experience pain in the hip, the knee, or both. These parts of the body can be an important part of sexual activity. Fatigue also can be a factor. If you're tired, you're going to be less interested in sexual activity.

What about drugs? Sexual problems may be caused by such medication as painkillers, sedatives, and tranquilizers, or by other types of drugs, including alcohol. It's true that small amounts of any of these may make you feel more relaxed (increasing the possibility of sex), but too much can work against you. The use of alcohol is notorious for reducing sexual ability.

Some drugs can have a direct effect on sexual desire. For example, certain medication (such as tranquilizers, which may be prescribed to reduce anxiety) can suppress sexual desire or decrease your ability to achieve orgasm. Antihypertensive (blood-pressure) medication and some antidepressants also can have an effect on sexual performance.

What about sex after joint replacement (or other) surgery? Sexual relationships can, in many cases, be resumed once healing has taken place. Many doctors recommend waiting at least six to eight weeks after major surgery before resuming intercourse. So make sure you consult your surgeon before resuming sexual relations.

The return to sex can be either extremely pleasurable or extremely disappointing, depending on each participant's point of view. If you were looking for skyrockets but were very nervous, you may have been disappointed. Inability to perform is not unusual following surgery, but it need not be permanent.

WHAT CAN YOU DO?

What can you do if your interest in sex has been affected by physical problems? Because painful movement or restriction of joints can make sex difficult, it's important to explore possible ways of changing this. Since movement can increase pain, you'll want to minimize your movement or try positions that require less activity on your part. Try using treatments that can help relax your muscles or reduce pain, such as moist heat, warm baths, or compresses. Limbering-up exercises may pave the way to more pleasurable sexual encounters. (This gives new meaning to the term "warm-up," doesn't it?)

Since sexual activity often takes place at night, acetaminophen, aspirin, or other painkilling medication may be taken before sexual encounters so that pain relief is at its maximum.

You may want to try different positions. Some of them may put less of a strain on painful or restricted joints. If sexual activity is painful, you may be better off taking a more passive and less active part in your encounters. In addition, on some occasions the use of simple devices such as pillows or knee pads can make sex a lot less painful.

Is there any particular time of day when you experience less pain? For some people, it may be too uncomfortable to have sex late at night. For others, the morning or the early part of the day may be the less desirable time. Working these problems out takes the cooperation of both partners. Children, work, and other responsibilities may interfere, of course, but it's better to have sex at planned times than not at all. Frequently, sexual problems can be helped by using your imagination and experimenting with variations in position, timing, and technique.

If pain or other symptoms are a problem, discuss this with your partner. Together, you may be able to come up with a solution, such as the use of a sexual position that removes pressure from the affected area. You can also use relaxation techniques (see Chapter 5) to help enhance the pleasures of sexual activities and decrease the pain.

A satisfying sexual relationship can actually help relieve pain. Not only is it distracting, but sexual stimulation and orgasm actually prompt the release of endorphins, those body chemicals that block pain and produce pleasure in the brain. What a pleasurable way to reduce pain!

There may be times that certain sexual activities just have to be put on hold. Actually, that may be an excellent idea. After all, just holding each other can be wonderful, too! So explore other ways to pleasure your partner and yourself. The twenty-second kiss can revive the feelings that brought you together. A long, slow, deliberate kiss—which need not progress to further sexual activity—can be a great reviver of closeness. The sixty-second hug is also wonderful to reconnect after a stressful day or when you are in pain. About halfway through a long hug, you will relax in each other's arms and feel a great release of tension.

Be patient. Don't feel that you have to accomplish everything at once. By minimizing the pressure you place on yourself, you can maximize enjoyment and get back into the swing of things at your own pace. Feel free to experiment with various techniques and activities to determine the degree of arousal that is safe and comfortable.

Psychological Problems

Your body isn't the only thing that may affect your sexual interest. Your mind also comes into the picture.

What's your most important sex organ? Think hard, now. The correct response is . . . your brain! So if a sexual problem has no physical basis, then its cause must be psychological. In fact, the psychological variables that affect sexual activity are just as real as physical factors. Anxiety, depression, and fear can all form emotional blocks that severely impair sexual enjoyment.

Let's look at various psychological problems that can affect your sex life and discuss how these obstacles can be overcome.

POOR SELF-IMAGE

Living with OA may affect your self-esteem. Do you feel like a different person? Do you like yourself less because of your condition? Do you feel "damaged"? Are you uncomfortable thinking about your partner looking at your body and seeing what OA has done to it? If your answer to any of these questions is yes, your self-esteem has suffered as a result of this disease.

Body image, an important component of self-esteem, plays a major role in one's sexuality. If you have a positive opinion of yourself, then your ability to respond to sex is positive. You are less likely to worry that your partner will reject or disapprove of your body. As a result, you may feel less need to limit your sexual activity simply to minimize this chance of rejection.

Self-consciousness can be a big problem. Some people with OA feel less feminine or masculine because of changes in the way they move or look. How has your condition affected your perception of your sexuality? If having OA makes you feel less sexually attractive (and this is not uncommon), then you've targeted an important area to work on. See what things you can change. For example, consider getting advice about clothes, makeup, and other appearance enhancers. And remember that nobody's perfect. Everybody has flaws. It makes sense to work on enhancing your looks in whatever ways are appropriate. After all, regardless of the problem, there are usually ways to improve things. But improving your mental attitude is just as important. For those problems that can't be modified, use some of the thought-changing procedures described earlier in Chapters 12, 13, and 14. They may be the key to your future happiness!

EMOTIONAL INTERFERENCE

Emotions can get in the way, too. Depression is well known to lower sexual interest as well as mood. You may be so withdrawn that you simply have no interest in relations. Anxiety concerning sex itself, the intimacy of your relationship, or your sexual performance can also hold you back.

Any of this can happen to anyone—not just to people with OA. Fortunately, it can also be changed with proper awareness, interaction, improved communication, and, if necessary, therapy.

If you don't currently have a sexual partner, it may be uncomfortable for you to even think about finding someone new, knowing the problems you're having with OA. Take things one step at a time. Be more social, look to make new friends, and try not to worry about the more intimate activities that might occur in the future.

FEAR OF PREGNANCY

Many people with OA develop the disease after their childbearing years have passed, but for some, OA begins earlier in life. If so, you may be afraid of getting pregnant. This fear can certainly interfere with sexual enjoyment. Even if you use a birth control, you may still be nervous, and this may make it hard for you to enjoy sex spontaneously. But sex does not have to be 100-percent spontaneous in order to be pleasurable. And perhaps there are additional things you can do to decrease your chances of pregnancy. Discuss these with your physician before moving into separate bedrooms!

Should You Conceive?

There are always plenty of question marks when it comes to deciding to have a child. If you are a woman with OA, there are even more than usual. What about your medication? What about selfishness or guilt feelings? Will you really be able to care for the baby if your OA makes it difficult to fasten a diaper or feed the little one? What about breast-feeding? Will your medication enter your milk and, in turn, your baby?

If you decide you do want to have a baby, will you have more difficulty conceiving because of OA? No—unless the pain and restricted mobility of your condition prevent you from having intercourse. Will osteoarthritis itself cause a difficult or unsafe pregnancy? It shouldn't. OA should not have any effect on pregnancy, although it may compound common pregnancy-related discomforts such as backache and fatigue. And all the other problems that can disrupt any normal pregnancy can still occur—such pleasures as morning sickness, swollen ankles, and mood swings.

The best thing to do is to bring all issues out into the open and discuss them—with your partner, your primary doctor, and your obstetrician/gynecologist. You should thoroughly discuss all questions about the feasibility of conceiving and bearing a child—as well as your use of medications and other ongoing treatment for OA during pregnancy—*before* you attempt to conceive.

If You Do Conceive

Pregnancy can place additional stress on you, although it is impossible to predict what will happen during anyone's pregnancy. Pregnancy shouldn't have any major long-range effects on your OA, either positive or negative. As a result, you will probably decide whether to attempt (or avoid) pregnancy for the same reasons that you would if you didn't have OA.

In general, it's usually a good idea to avoid most medications during pregnancy. But this is not always possible. Tylenol and aspirin, for example, have been used by many women during their pregnancies, without any damage to the fetus. Of course, you should make sure to check with your physician if you have any questions. In all cases, don't take decisions regarding medication and pregnancy lightly. And, even more important, don't take decisions into your own hands, but work with your doctor. That's what you have a doctor for, right?

If OA is affecting your hips, you should take this into consideration when preparing for childbirth. A caesarian section may be necessary if you are unable to get into birth positions.

Otherwise, pregnancy should not be more of a problem for you than for anyone else, especially if you have a mild case of OA. The keys to a successful pregnancy are awareness, appropriate medical supervision, and careful planning. Take all these factors into consideration, and then—good luck!

WHAT CAN YOU DO?

If any psychological problems are affecting your sexual desire or performance, you will want to get to the root cause and use coping strategies to eliminate the troubling emotions. For instance, let's say you know that OA has made you feel less sexual and that this is causing problems. You have now targeted an important area on which to work. Recognize how your thinking plays a role in determining the way you feel. Why is it that you are feeling less sexual? Is it because of the pain, or because of the way your self-image has been affected? Do what you can to improve your thinking and increase your feelings of self-esteem. Focus on your good qualities. Concentrate on the overall enjoyment you can derive from intimacy.

If anxiety or depression is affecting your sexual well-being, you'll want to improve your attitude and combat the troubling emotion. Use some of the thought-changing procedures described earlier in the book. They may be the key to your future happiness!

A very important part of sexual relationships is communication. If you and your partner can share thoughts and feelings, you'll be in much better shape to work out any sexual problems that may occur as a result of your condition. It is important to discuss sexual problems with your partner. If communication problems exist, difficulties may be very hard to resolve.

What might you talk about with your partner? Acknowledge and discuss any sexual fears or problems, such as pain with certain positions. If necessary, work to alter the ways in which the two of you express your sexual desires. Fully communicate your needs. For instance, if there are times when you're in too much pain or just too tired for sexual activity, tell your partner honestly how you feel. Talk about what feels good and what hurts during sex.

Besides communicating your feelings and fears to your partner, you might also want to discuss any problems with your physician or other health-care professionals. A qualified sex therapist who understands OA may be helpful for some couples. You can also take your partner with you to the doctor and talk about the problem openly and honestly.

Everything that's been said in this section assumes that your sexual interest or performance has been affected by physical or psychological problems, and that your partner is suffering as a result. But what if the opposite is true? What if you still have normal sexual desires and abilities, but your partner is the one who's afraid or thinks sexual activity may create additional problems? Perhaps your partner sees you as being fragile simply because you have OA, and is reluctant to initiate or respond to sexual overtures. Discuss this together. Make sure that you communicate with each other, and then establish ground rules so that you know which sexual activities are okay and which, if any, aren't. And if these one-on-one attempts at solving problems aren't successful, don't hesitate to get some professional assistance. The results will be well worth the effort.

And Now the Climax

When dealing with any sexual problems resulting from your OA, remember that there are many ways to improve both your feelings regarding sex and your enjoyment of various sexual activities. Psychological coping strategies can help you overcome many obstacles related to interest in sex and enjoyment of sexual activity. But the most important intervention is open communication with your partner. Even if your sex life becomes less active, you can still have a warm relationship—but you can't if there are bitter feelings and misgivings. Honest discussions, marked by understanding, are a vital part of coping with sexual problems, just as they are a necessary part of coping with any other aspect of OA.

Remember: Having OA doesn't mean that sexual activity must be reduced, curtailed, or totally eliminated. It can still be as pleasurable and as important as the partners want it to be.

CHAPTER TWENTY-SIX

Living with Someone Who Has Osteoarthritis

A medical problem such as osteoarthritis doesn't affect just the person with the disease. It also affects everyone who is close to that person. Those who are in the inner circle, and especially those in the immediate family, are affected in the most significant way. They are also in the best position to help.

Illness can create troubling changes in relationships. No kidding! If you live with someone who has OA, you may have a number of concerns. You may now view that person—and even yourself—differently. Maybe you see the person as being more fragile. Maybe you are reminded of your own vulnerability. Maybe you used to depend on that person, and now you have to shoulder more responsibilities.

What does all this mean? First, you have legitimate concerns. Although you share the concerns of the individual who has osteoarthritis, you also worry about yourself. Concerns about the future, your loved one's health, and financial issues may all be troublesome to you.

This chapter will first explain what you can do to help your loved one. It will then outline some ways that you can help yourself cope with the problems involved in living with someone who has OA.

How You Can Help Someone with OA

If you are close to someone with OA, you have an important responsibility, with many components. But what exactly is your job, and how can you best perform it? Read on!

BECOME A LOYAL LEARNER

You can help your loved one a great deal simply by learning as much as you can about osteoarthritis and its treatment. The knowledge you obtain will allow you to provide support and true understanding. Both can offer tremendous support to someone with OA. Knowing the facts may help you as well, as it may dissipate any fear of the unknown and help eliminate your confusion over symptoms or treatments.

MAINTAIN NORMALCY

When spending time with your loved one, try to behave as you always have. Try to minimize any changes in your interactions. I don't mean to suggest that you should ignore, through word or deed, the osteoarthritis. As we will discuss later on in the chapter, it's vital to be open about feelings, and to honestly discuss any problems. Just try not to dwell on your loved one's condition.

Why is it so important to maintain normalcy? Well, having to deal with OA is unpleasant enough, and worries about the way in which the condition will change everyday life can also be upsetting. So by keeping life as normal as possible, you will help to compensate for any changes that must take place.

ENCOURAGE, DON'T PESTER

Certainly, you should encourage your loved one to adhere to proper treatment routines. But don't badger. If the person is not taking proper care of herself, there is a limit to what you can do to change her behavior. Yelling usually doesn't help (and it can hurt your vocal cords).

If your loved one is not taking care of herself, should you tell her physician? That's a hard question to answer. You don't want to overstep your bounds and be resented. At the same time, you don't want to sit back and watch unnecessary problems develop. This is especially true if the person doesn't seem to care.

So what should you do? Play it by ear. Voice your concerns, explaining that you're afraid of any problems becoming worse due to lack of treatment. Then listen carefully to your loved one's response before deciding whether to contact her physician or take other action.

PROVIDE SUPPORT, NOT PITY

Because of the difficulties of living with OA and its treatment, you may sympathize with your loved one. You may feel sad about what he has to go through. The sympathy you feel may help you provide beneficial support. But don't pity him, as this can be destructive.

Be aware that symptoms of—and treatment for—OA can affect mood, causing depression, anxiety, and other emotional reactions. Try to prepare yourself, and resist any temptation to separate yourself. OA is not contagious, of course, and your loving support may be one of the most important factors in your loved one's emotional state. How, exactly, can you help? If you sense that your loved one is wallowing in self-pity, you may be able to help by just being there, reaching out, and touching. Sometimes, just by listening and allowing feelings to be expressed, you can turn negative emotions into positive ones. Don't feel that you have to quickly snap your loved one out of any depression. A certain amount of self-pity can be a necessary self-indulgence. Problems arise only when the period of self-pity continues for too long a time. If this happens, do what you can to restore spirits, consulting a professional if necessary.

During times of depression, you will probably want to be as encouraging as possible. But avoid giving your loved one false hope or making false promises. It's not always wonderfully reassuring to hear that "everything will be fine; the pain will go away." On occasion, this comment can cause more harm than good by causing a loss of faith in your honesty and candor.

What if your loved one is in so much pain or is so fatigued that he can do little or nothing? At such times, it is not appropriate for you to insist that the person "get up and do something." That won't help the situation. Instead, try to help out by taking over some of the existing obligations and responsibilities. This may help reduce some of the pressure, and will allow your loved one to conserve his energy. At the same time, don't allow your loved one to baby himself. In general, if he is able to do something— even if it takes some time—permit it. If you feel that the person is malingering, by all means discuss it. Try to make life as normal as possible.

AVOID OVERPROTECTIVENESS

As a family member or close friend, it's very important to tune in to the needs of your loved one. Don't assume that you should be overprotective or underprotective simply because that's the way you would want others to act if you were ill. Be sure to find out what your loved one wants, and try, as much as possible, to act accordingly.

Don't pressure your special someone. Sure, you want to be supportive. When she is tired, for instance, you'll want to relieve her of some chores or other responsibilities. But provide sufficient space for her to regain some control over her own life. How? When she is no longer tired, be sure to permit the resumption of normal activities. Don't tell her to get into bed and rest. Have faith in your loved one. If she really doesn't feel well, rest will be the order of the day. Otherwise, back off.

What about accompanying your loved one on visits to the doctor? If she agrees, you may want to go along for the ride—both to offer support and to lend another set of ears. There may be times when the doctor might want to discuss something with you. It might be a good idea for four ears rather than two ears to listen when the doctor is explaining OA, medication, or other aspects of the treatment program. However, if the person wants to go alone and feels strongly about it, don't force the issue.

What's the bottom line? Work with your loved one to set ground rules as soon as possible. Hopefully, she will initiate this. If not, you can start the discussion. Talk about your interest in being as supportive as possible, and ask what you can do to help. Things will move more smoothly once you have a good idea of what to do and when to do it. Even if no clear-cut answers emerge, at least you'll share some constructive communication, which will lay the groundwork for handling future problems. Perhaps most important—and, possibly, most difficult—try to respect the decisions made regarding how she wants things handled. Discussions are fine, but you shouldn't be the one making the final decisions.

KEEP TALKING!

What's the best way to talk to your loved one? Unfortunately, because everybody's different and because needs change along with moods and circumstances, there's no way to know for sure. At certain times, you may feel that it's best to respond with sympathy and understanding. At other times, it may be best to just ignore the situation and walk away. To a degree, you'll have to play things by ear, remaining as attuned to your loved one as possible.

However you decide to talk, by all means, *keep talking!* The most important key to maintaining family harmony is communication. Perhaps you have always communicated effectively, even before the pain and other problems of OA entered your life. If so, you're among the lucky ones. If not, it's imperative to establish the lines of communication and keep them open.

Why is good communication so important? Only through communication will you learn how your loved one feels, both physically and emotionally. And only by knowing this will you be able to help. This doesn't mean that the conversations will always be pleasant. Talking about treatment problems, depression, fears, or pain isn't very enjoyable, especially if you don't have any solutions. But with good communication, any difficulties will be outweighed by the feeling of closeness that results from shared experiences and concerns.

As much as you would like to talk to your loved one, there may be times when he or she is unwilling to do that. When this happens, it's perfectly okay to be reassuring that you're aware of this lack of desire to talk right now, but that you'll be there when a sympathetic ear is needed.

Sometimes you may feel that it would be helpful to ask your loved one how *you* can cope with the difficulty of the situation—with the uncertainties you feel, and your own fears about this condition. There's certainly nothing wrong with pointing out that you're concerned. Make sure you do it at an appropriate time, though. And if you see that the subject is upsetting your loved one, put the conversation on hold.

Take Care of Yourself, Too!

Although you probably learned a great deal about the experience of OA from reading this book, so far we have paid little attention to the problems that OA poses for the caregivers. There are moments when a family member has a harder time dealing with this condition than does the person who has it! You may feel many of the same emotions experienced by the person with OA, but feel more helpless and out of control because everything is happening *around* you rather than *to* you. In addition, as a caregiver, you will encounter special problems of your own. Let's take a look at some of the problems you may face, and see how you can care not only for your loved one, but also for an equally important person—yourself.

GUILT

In Chapter 17, we discussed how your loved one may experience feelings of guilt as a result of having OA. You, too, may be troubled by this emotion. You may feel (irrationally) that you somehow contributed to the OA. You might think that you should have been more insistent about a doctor being seen when problems first occurred. You may feel guilty because, although you are concerned about your loved one, you resent the fact that this condition is going to interfere with the quality of *your* life. This can make you feel especially bad, because your anger and resentment are directed toward somebody who may appear to be vulnerable and, of course, is suffering.

How can you cope with your feelings of guilt? Work to restructure your own thinking, just as your loved one who experiences guilt must do the same thing. Keep reminding yourself that you did not cause the OA. You are not a bad person. You are doing what you can to help. By reworking your negative thoughts, you will be able to reduce any feelings of guilt that might arise. (For more about coping with guilt, see Chapter 17.)

DEPRESSION

Just as your loved one will sometimes feel depressed, you too may sometimes experience depression. This can result from a number of things, including lifestyle changes. Accept that it's okay to feel this way. After all, it's certainly depressing when life's patterns have to change because of a chronic illness. However, don't allow this feeling to linger. Find a technique that will help to lift the depression.

Again, begin by restructuring your thinking. Depression is often caused by negative thoughts, so you'll want to follow the guidelines for changing them provided in Chapters 12 through 14. In addition, be sure to reserve some time each day for yourself. You need to find a time when you can do the things you enjoy. This isn't being selfish or negligent. Rather, by helping yourself, you'll be making yourself stronger and better able to support your loved one.

THE LONG VERSUS THE SHORT OF IT

When someone experiences an acute (short-term) medical problem—such as pneumonia, an infection, or a broken bone—it may be easy for friends and relatives to rally around, provide support and understanding, and temporarily take over responsibilities. But a condition such as OA is a different matter. There will be times when your loved one may be able to do very little, and you will have to take on many more chores. At other times, she will be able to take on more tasks and resume normal activities. These ups and downs can create major problems. And the fact that there is no definite end in sight will not make your adjustment any easier.

How can you cope with problems caused by the chronic nature of OA? Once again, work on your thinking. Long-range worries lead to long-term unhappiness. So instead of thinking about the future, do what you can each day to support your loved one, and to make all of your lives as full and happy as possible. Have faith in your ability to rise to new challenges if and when it becomes necessary to do so.

A FINAL NOTE ON SELF-CARE

You know that someone with OA needs care and support. But don't ignore the fact that you, too, need—and deserve—nurturing and caring attention. Don't be afraid to reach out and get it. Don't feel that, because you're not the person who is sick, you have to take a backseat. Your emotions can suffer as well. Remember that you can benefit from the same kinds of support groups as your loved one does. Don't hesitate to take advantage of the many resources available. To continue to be at your best for yourself, for your loved one, and for other family members, you need to be strong.

A Supportive Conclusion

True, OA is not affecting your body. But it is certainly affecting your life in other ways. By following the suggestions in this chapter, you can help yourself become stronger, more emotionally stable, and more supportive of your loved one. After all, she is not the only one who has to cope with OA!

On to the Future

Well, you've just about finished this book. We've covered a lot of information about osteoarthritis. Tremendous progress has been made in the quest for new, more effective medications, surgical procedures and other interventions. Ongoing research continues to investigate the ways that joints function, as well as techniques that may decrease damage to bones and tissues and improve bone growth and repair. These will all serve to further improve the quality of life for people who suffer from OA.

Perhaps by the time you read this, some drug or treatment may have proven even more successful than the ones discussed in this book. For example, recent research has been investigating drugs that may stimulate cartilage regeneration, drugs that inhibit the enzymes that are involved in the process of cartilage degeneration, and the potential for cartilage transplantation. It remains to be seen what new developments may improve your life with OA. But it's very reassuring that many experts continue to search for ways to help the millions of people who suffer.

Although it would be impossible to discuss every conceivable problem related to OA in this book, I hope that what you've read will help you to develop your own strategies for coping. Because things change, and something that troubles you one day may not trouble you the next (and vice versa), use this book as a resource. Whenever you have questions about how to cope with a certain aspect of osteoarthritis, consult the appropriate section. If you have any comments, information that you believe is important, or additional questions, feel free to write to me in care of Avery Books, Penguin Putnam, Inc., 375 Hudson Street, New York, NY 10014. I'd be happy to hear from you.

And so, as I said at the very beginning of the book, until such time as there is no longer a medical condition called osteoarthritis, keep on coping the best you can. Look brightly ahead, act proudly, and enjoy life as best you can. Remember that—despite osteoarthritis—you can *always* improve the quality of your life!

For Further Reading

The following books—which provide more information on the material presented in this book, and focus on other topics as well—may help you cope with various aspects of living with osteoarthritis. But by no means should you limit yourself to those listed below. Many other books and publications also examine osteoarthritis treatment, nutrition, the challenges of living with chronic illness, and other subjects that may be of interest to you. Don't hesitate to take advantage of all the information available at your local library or bookstore, from professional associations and support groups, and on the Internet.

Achterberg, Jeanne, Barbara Dossey, and Leslie Kolkmeier. *Rituals of Healing: Using Imagery for Health and Wellness.* New York: Bantam Doubleday Dell, 1994.

Balch, James F., and Phyllis A. Balch. *Prescription for Nutritional Healing,* 2nd Ed. Garden City Park, NY: Avery Publishing Group, 1997.

Butler, Robert, and Myrna Lewis. *Love and Sex After Forty.* New York: Harper and Row Publishers, 1986.

Fanning, Patrick. *Visualization for Change*. Oakland, CA: New Harbinger Publications, 1988.

Goldberg, Burton. *Alternative Medicine: The Definitive Guide*. Tiburon, CA: Future Medicine Publishing, Inc., 1998.

Lazarus, Arnold A. *In the Mind's Eye: The Power of Imagery for Personal Enrichment*. New York: Rawson Associates, 1984.

Linchitz, Richard M. *Life Without Pain*. Reading, MA: Addison-Wesley Publishing Co., Inc., 1988.

Lininger, Schuyler W., Alan R. Gaby, Steve Austin, Donald J. Brown, Jonathan V. Wright, and Jamie Miller. *The Natural Pharmacy: Complete Home Reference to Natural Medicine*. Rocklin, CA: Prima Publishing, 1999.

Phillips, Robert H. *Control Your Pain!: 169 Painless Strategies for Taking Charge of Your Body*. New York: Balance, 1996.

Simonton, Stephanie Matthews, and Robert L. Shook. *The Healing Family: The Simonton Approach for Families Facing Illness*. New York: Bantam Books, 1984.

Sobel, Dava, and Arthur C. Klein. *Arthritis: What Exercises Work*. New York: St. Martin's Press, 1995.

Theodosakis, Jason, Brenda Adderly, and Barry Fox. *The Arthritis Cure*. New York: St. Martin's Press, 1997.

Resource Groups

The following groups can provide you with more information on OA, suggest helpful books and videos, direct you to support groups, and inform you of other valuable services. Feel free to contact these organizations and benefit from their expertise.

Academy for Guided Imagery
P.O. Box 2070
Mill Valley, CA 94942
800-726-2070; 415-389-9324
http://www.interactiveimagery.com

American Academy of Pain
Management
13947 Mono Way #A
Sonora, CA 95370
209-533-9744
http://www.aapainmanage.org

American Chronic Pain
Association
P.O. Box 850

Rocklin, CA 95677
916-632-0922
http://www.theacpa.org

American College of Rheumatology
1800 Century Place, Suite 250
Atlanta, GA 30345
404-633-3777
http://www.rheumatology.org

American Massage Therapy
Association
820 Davis Street, Suite 100
Evanston, IL 60201
847-864-0123
http://www.amtamassage.org

American Society of Clinical
Hypnosis
130 East Elm Court, Suite 201
Roselle, IL 60172-2000
630-980-4740
http://www.asch.net

Arthritis Care
18 Stephenson Way
London NW1 2HD
England
020-7380-6500
http://www.arthritiscare.org.uk

Arthritis Foundation
National Office
1330 West Peachtree Street
Atlanta, GA 30309
800-283-7800; 404-872-7100
http://www.arthritis.org

Arthritis Society
National Office
393 University Avenue, Suite 1700
Toronto, Ontario M5G 1E6
Canada
800-321-1433; 416-979-7228
http://www.arthritis.ca

Association for Applied
Psychophysiology and Biofeedback
10200 West 44th Avenue,
Suite 304
Wheat Ridge, CO 80033

303-422-8436
http://www.aapb.org

National Chronic Pain Outreach
Association
P.O. Box 274
Millboro VA 24460
540-862-9437
E-mail: ncpoa@cfw.com

National Guild of Hypnotists
P.O. Box 308
Merrimack, NH 03054
603-429-9438
http://www.ngh.net

National Institute of Arthritis
and Musculoskeletal and
Skin Diseases
Building 31, Room 4C05
31 Center Drive, MSC 2350
Bethesda, MD 20892-2350
301-496-8190
http://www.nih.gov/niams

NCCAM Clearinghouse
National Center for Complemen-
tary and Alternative Medicine
National Institutes of Health
P.O. Box 8218
Silver Spring, MD 20907
888-644-6226
http://nccam.nih.gov

Index